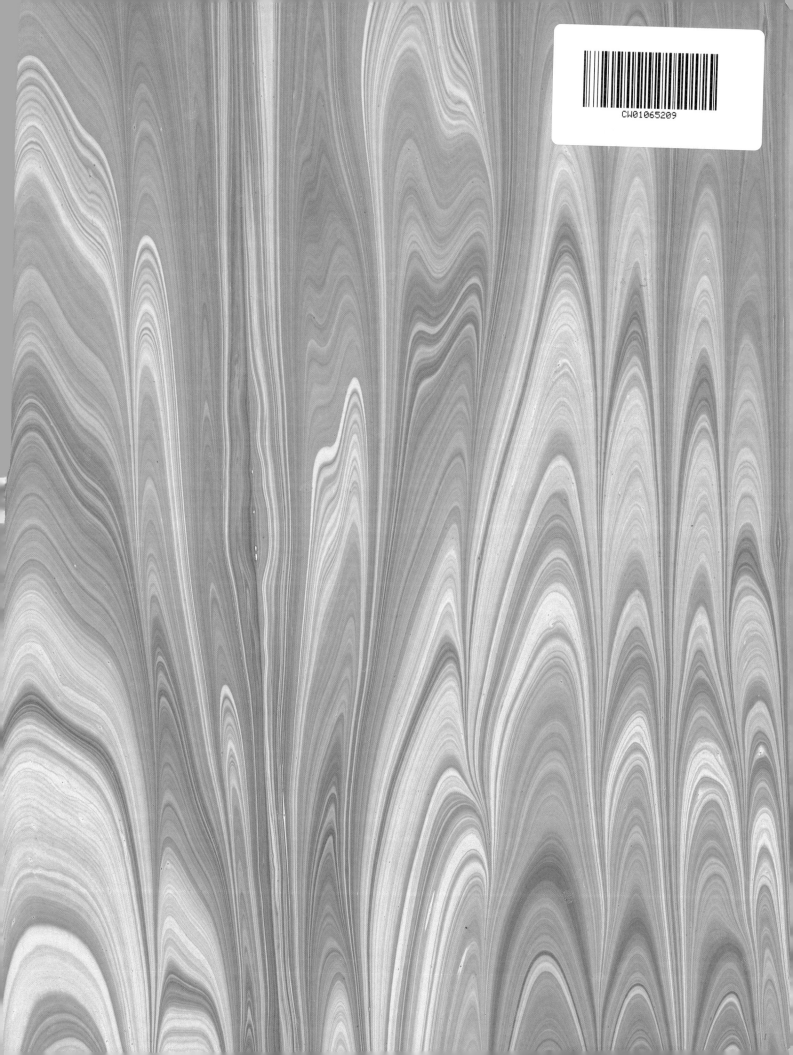

The Shaving Mug & Barber Bottle Book

Keith E. Estep

with value guide

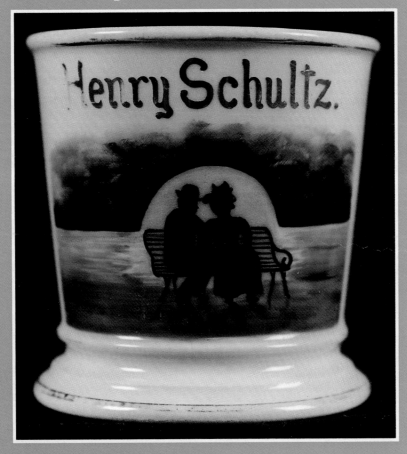

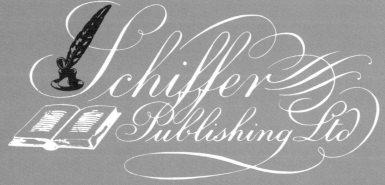

77 Lower Valley Road, Atglen, PA 19310

Dedication

This book is dedicated to my mother, Lois N. Estep, to my son, Colin D. Estep, and to my daughter, Kristin E. Estep.

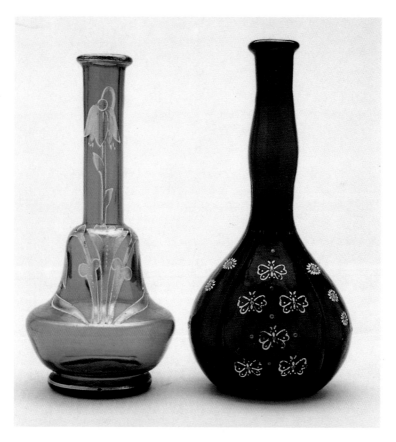

Left, green with gold art nouveau design. Right, amethyst with butterfly decoration.

Copyright © 1995 by Keith E. Estep.

All rights reserved. No part of this work may be reproduced or used in any forms or by any means–graphic, electronic or mechanical, including photocopying or information storage and retrieval systems–without written permission from the copyright holder.

Printed in Hong Kong.

Library of Congress Cataloging-in-Publication Data

Estep, Keith E.
   The shaving mug & barber bottle book, with value guide/Keith E. Estep.
      p.   cm.
   Includes index.
   ISBN: 0-88740-761-7
   1. Shaving mugs--United States--Collectors and collecting--Catalogs. 2. Barber bottles--United States--Collectors and collecting--Catalogs. I. Title. II. Title: Shaving mug and barber bottle book, with value guide.
NK4695.S5E88 1995
738.3'0973'075--dc20   94-44836
                          CIP

Title Page:
Moonlight, man and woman on bench. *Courtesy of Morris Pickerell, Jr.*

Published by Schiffer Publishing, Ltd.
77 Lower Valley Road
Atglen, PA 19310
Please write for a free catalog.
This book may be purchased from the publisher.
Please include $2.95 postage.
Try your bookstore first.

We are interested in hearing from authors
with book ideas on related subjects.

Contents

Acknowledgments

I wish to thank the people who helped me in preparing this book. They provided photographs of beautiful mugs and bottles, and invaluable information about this wonderful field of collecting. My gratitude goes to;

Michael J. Griffin, White Plains, New York
Anthony Gugliotti, Wolcott, Connecticut
Dr. Ralph Nix D.D.S., Red Bay, Alabama
Morris Pickerell, Jr., Ocala, Florida
Thomas and Penelope Nader
Ray and Theresa Jones
David Giese, Stafford, Virginia

Bernard Lukco, Springfield, Ohio
William and Phyllis Gilmore, Lancaster, Ohio
Roland F. Porter, Hinsdale, Illinois
Charles F. Kalb, Lady Lake, Florida
Mrs. Fred Willman
Julius Marymore
Mr. and Mrs. Frank Burton
and other collectors who wish
    to remain anonymous.

Without your support and assistance, this project would have been impossible.

Photo Credits

Robert Lawson, Hamden, Connecticut.
Fred Ortoli Photography, Seymour, Connecticut.
Photography by Elizabth Stemrich, Allentown, Pennsylvania.

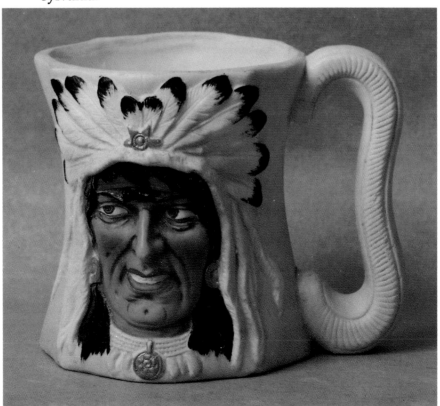

Raised design, Indian.

Foreword

Personalized shaving mugs of barber supply catalog quality are what collectors want and what drives this exciting, interesting hobby. I will concentrate my efforts on these items.

My collection started with my great-grandfather's mug about fifteen years ago. Since then I have built an advanced collection and have become a dealer as well. I have made some mistakes along the way, selling too cheap, buying too high, and passing on mugs I should have bought. This book will help to educate and inform others so they don't encounter the same problems.

I wish to thank the kindness of many first and second generation collectors who have shared their knowledge and opinions to me over the years. As one generation teaches the next, this hobby will continue to bring pleasure to those who pursue it.

I write this book to help the collector, dealer, and those persons that wish to sell their mugs. It grows out of my years of experience as a collector and a dealer in shaving mugs and barbershop memorabilia. In my business I buy and sell shaving mugs and barber bottles, provide collection assistance and management advice to my clients, and provide private treaty sales and appraisals. If some questions arise or an area seems gray, OLD LYME MUGS will be at your service. Contact me by writing or calling:

Keith Estep
OLD LYME MUGS
P.O. Box 4118
Old Lyme, CT 06371
203-434-9244

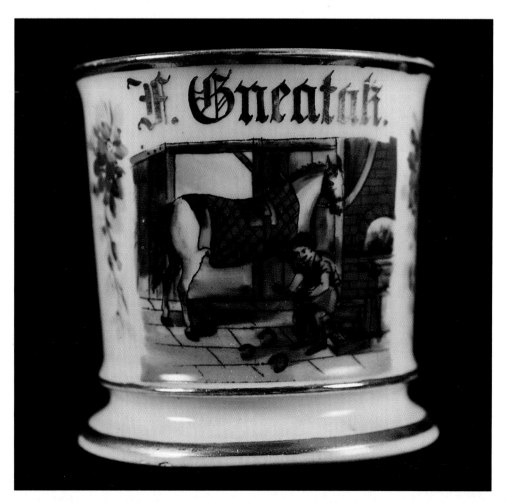

Blacksmith working. *Courtesy of Morris Pickerell, Jr.*

Introduction

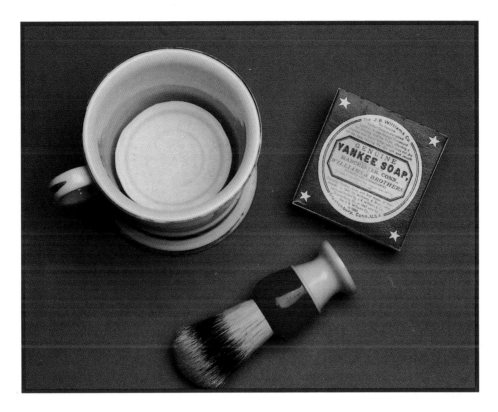

The shaving mug is nothing more than a container designed to hold a bar of shaving soap. It was a functional item which saw daily use. For decades the barber would use one mug to provide the lather for all his customers. Then, in the 1870s, a fungus known as *Barber's Itch* gave birth to the personalized shaving mug. This affliction was irritating enough that any shop known to have the problem was carefully avoided, possibly forcing the barber out of business. To avoid this fate, barbers encouraged their customers to have their own, sanitary, personal shaving mug.

To encourage the purchase of mugs, someone had the idea of having an individual's name, in gold script, on his mug. These mugs were imported from Europe and were made of high quality china. The mugs were decorated at the barber's supply distributor. The barber would receive a commission on any mug that a customer ordered.

Thus began the shaving mug era. It can be divided into three periods. From the 1870s to 1891 was the early stage, when the idea of personalized mugs slowly spread. From 1891 to 1914 was the golden age of mugs, a time of high artistry and great popularity. The period from 1914 to the 1920s was the decline, when the safety razor began its entry into the market place and shaving entered the privacy of one's own home.

These years were the age of great immigration to the United States. Many came to this country with little more than the shirt on their back. They lived in squalid tenements, where indoor plumbing and running water was a luxury. The barber shop provided baths as well as shaves and haircuts. Many of these shops were ethnic, providing a haven for the immigrant, where he could be among friends and speak his native language. For many the barber shop became a social gathering place, as a customer would visit the shop frequently, often on a daily basis.

Many immigrants were illiterate. Having a mug with a name on it would have no value. It may have been the barber who first saw the need for a mug with an illustration of a trade design, to provide this customer with a mug with which he could identify. By the 1880s the major barber shop distributors all had decorating departments which provided trade design illustrations on mugs. Highly decorative floral design and fraternal emblem mugs were also produced.

To provide quality illustrations there was a need for china decorators. Most of these men learned their trade in Europe, and the majority, I believe, were of German origin. Perhaps some of them were enticed to this country with the promise of immediate employment. The trade design decoration of mugs, although unique to the United States and Canada, was very similar to their trade in the old country. As a result mug artistry improved greatly with their arrival.

The golden years started in 1891, that year the McKinley tariff forced all imported items to have a country of origin stamp. The mugs of this era have marks on the bottom such as "T" & "V" Limoges, "J" & "C" Bavaria, Leonard Vienna, Austria, etc. Some mugs had the word "Germany" incised in the base of the mug. These stamp marks are usually green in color. Some of the major barber suppliers would also stamp the bottom of the mug with their logo. Some examples of the distributor's stamp are "Aug. Kern" of St. Louis, "Herold Bros." of Cleveland and "Eugene Berninghaus" of Cincinnati, Ohio. Very few mugs bear the stamp or signature of the artists themselves. Of the few artists did put their name on the base, one was J.R.. Voldan.

These golden years from 1891-1914 had the finest artistry and decoration. Some illustrations have photographic realism and some are so finely rendered that you need a magnifying glass to see and appreciate all the details. The gold trim that flanked the illustration, called the cartouch, was the most elaborate of any period in the mug era.

More mugs were produced during this period than any other. I would say that 60% to 75% of all mugs in collections today are from this era.

The period of decline started about 1914. There is a noticeable lessening in the artistic quality of the mugs, which seem to have less detail and clarity. Perhaps the old German mug decorators were reaching the age of retirement. The quality of the mug itself declined, as well. World War disrupted the flow of quality mugs to this country. While America was involved in the production of mugs, they didn't have the quality of the European china. America also produced a semi-vitreous mug. This was not china but a glazed pottery similar to kitchen mixing bowls. The artistry on these mugs often is sloppy and appears to be cartoon-like.

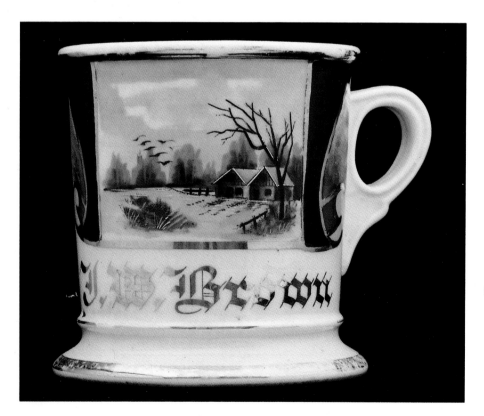

Cabins. *Courtesy of Anthony Gugliotti.*

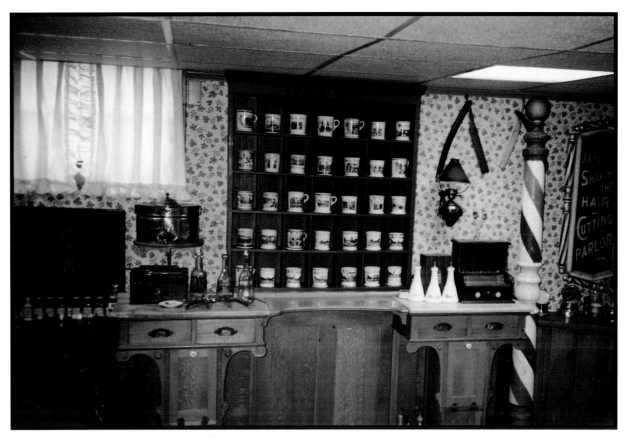

In 1917 America entered the war. All soldiers and sailors were issued a Gillette safety razor. After learning to shave themselves there was no reason to pay a barber to do it. This one factor alone caused a rapid decline in mug era.

After the war, mugs were still available but they were no longer a profitable retail item. Many barber suppliers shut down their mug decorating departments. Mugs were still produced during the 1920s and some of these have very rare graphics, such as airplanes and advanced autos.

As the mug era died some mugs went home with their owners, some were thrown away, and some retreated to barber shop basements and were forgotten. But a few people started to collect them. Barbers had the easiest access. Others may have had an interest in their own occupations, like the undertaker who traveled to various barber shops in search of "Hearse" and "Coffin" mugs, offering to pay 50 cents or a dollar. Great collections were established and it was cheap.

In 1949 the first book about mugs was published, *Occupational Shaving Mugs*, by W. Porter Ware. This book helped to set prices for collectible mugs. The most expensive mug was "make own price above $25."[1]

The 1950s saw the rise of the first generation collectors. These people, armed with Porter Ware's book, built their own great collections. Many original owners of mugs were dying off, and mugs were plentiful. The cost was $10 or $15. During the 1960s the price of mugs started to escalate. Sometimes a price of $50 or $100 was paid.

In 1972 a second book was published, *Antique Shaving Mugs of the United States*, by Robert Blake Powell. This is a great book on the subject of barbering and shaving mugs. After this book the second generation of collectors came along. During the 1970s good mugs started to bring $100-$200 at auctions. In 1978 Blake Powell published his second book, *Occupational and Fraternal Shaving Mugs of the United States*. Many collectors submitted photos of their collections for this book.

In 1980, a group of fourteen collectors founded the "National Shaving Mug Collectors Association". At this writing it has 450 members and I have the honor to stand as vice president of this organization.

The "NSMCA" meets twice a year and issues a quarterly newsletter. Membership is $15 a year. The enjoyment and education is well worth the dues.

In writing this book I find it necessary to provide certain details of collecting, because mugs of good quality now sell for several hundred and sometimes thousands of dollars.

A new generation of collectors seems to spring up after the publication of a book. I hope a third generation comes along after this one.

Chapter 1
Collector's Terms

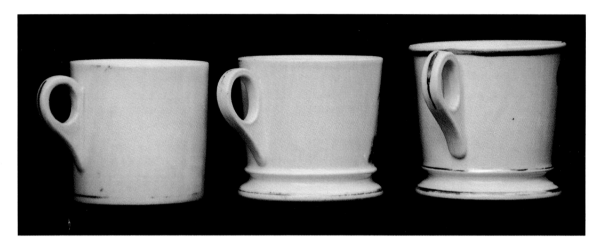

The three distinctive patterns of shaving mugs. Left to right:
the straight blank, the short blank, and the standard blank.

Collectors use certain terms when describing mugs.

The Blank. This refers to the size and shape of the mug, not the illustration. Blanks range in size from 3 1/4 to 4 inches. There are three distinctive patterns of mugs.

1. The "straight" or "shapeless" blank is usually 3 1/4 inches. It was used throughout the mug years, but primarily pre-1891.

Shaving mugs ranged in size from 3 1/4" to 4".

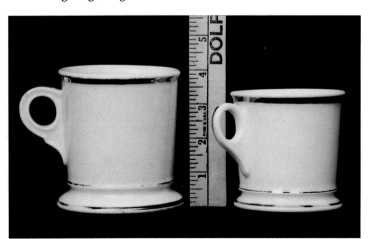

2. The "short" or "early" blanks are 3 1/4 inches. They were used exclusively in the pre-1891 years. They have three characteristics:
   a. The lip or top of the mug ends straight.
   b. The base has no country of origin stamp or mark.
   c. A flat gold of high quality was used for names and trim.
3. The standard blank was made in all sizes, but the most common is 3 5/8 inches. This blank was used from 1891 till the end. These mugs also have three characteristics:
   a. The lip is rounded
   b. The base has country of origin stamp and sometimes supply distributor and artist stamp.
   c. The use of mirror finish gold.

There is also an American blank known as semi-vitreous, which is part pottery. These come mainly in a 3 1/2 or 3 3/4 inch size. They have a crackling glaze similar to early kitchen bowls. Many of these mugs bear the stamp "Royal International China".

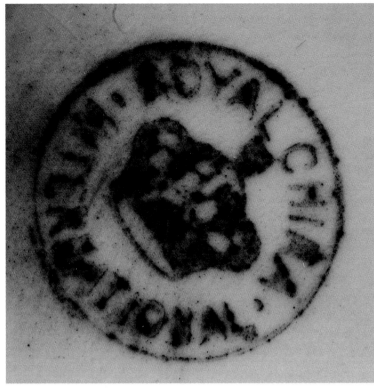

Royal International China stamp.

The Wrap. This refers to the color of the non-illustrated portion of the mug. There are three types of wraps.

Complete Wrap This covers the entire mug's graphic area. This is used to highlight graphics that are gold. It can also highlight light colored graphics.

Standard Wrap This covers the mug except for the illustration field. The common colors are dark red, blue and green.

Half Wrap This covers the top half area of the mug. This usually has an arch over the illustration or name.

The wrap is a nice touch, but, with one exception, it doesn't add value. The one wrap that collectors seek is a complete black wrap on a good Fraternal or Occupational mug. Some advanced collectors have racks reserved for these types of mugs. If a mug is rare, it would be much more rare as a black wrap. Floral and entry mugs have little or no extra value being black wrapped.

Sometimes a new black wrap is applied to an old mug. This is an attempt to cover up an old side illustration, with a fake illustration of a rare subject applied to the mug. Inspect all mugs closely before buying.

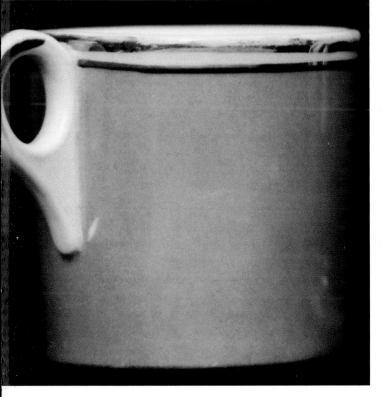

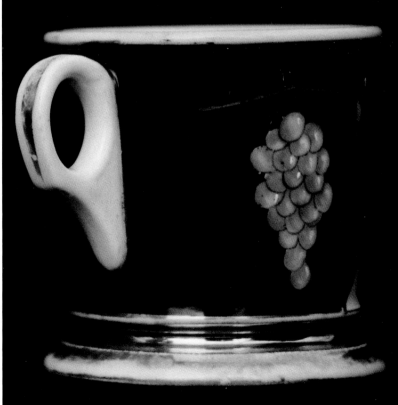

The complete wrap.

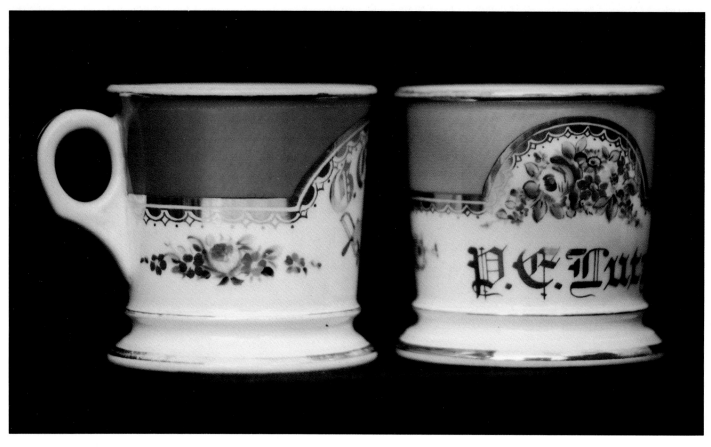

The half wrap.

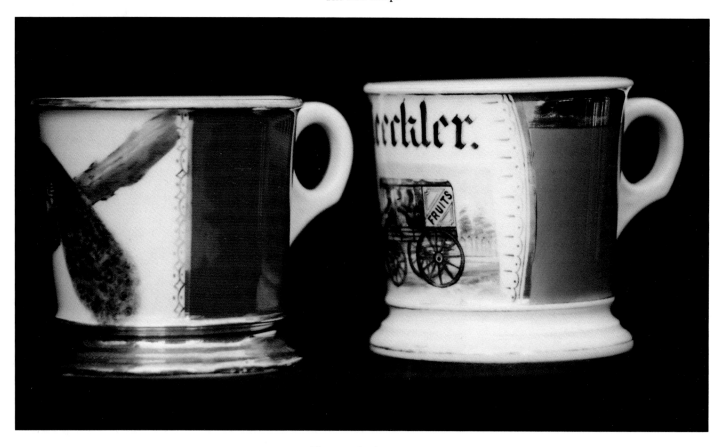

The standard wrap.

Gold. All names and trim are real gold. There are two types of gold on mugs. The first is the old dull finish variety. This type appears on early blanks, from about 1870 to about 1885. This seems to be the more durable type, since in many cases these older mugs have less gold wear than the newer mirror finish gold. The second type appears on all mugs from 1891 on. It has a bright mirror finish.

I have placed an old $20 gold piece next to both types of gold. The gold coin is 90% pure. As you can see, it has the same color as the gold finish on the old style mugs. As gold was the most expensive item it is reasonable to assume that the new mirror finish gold was of a less expensive grade.

Gothic letters in gold was the most common form of placing names on mugs. This is referred to in the old catalogs as "old English text". Other types you will find are gold block letters, black script, black block letters, and black gothic with gold highlights.

Sometimes you may find a mug with the name worn. After a few years of heavy use the name could be completely gone. This is because the name was the last graphic to be put on the mug. And it would only be fired once. As this was the weakest point of the mug, it would be the first to show wear.

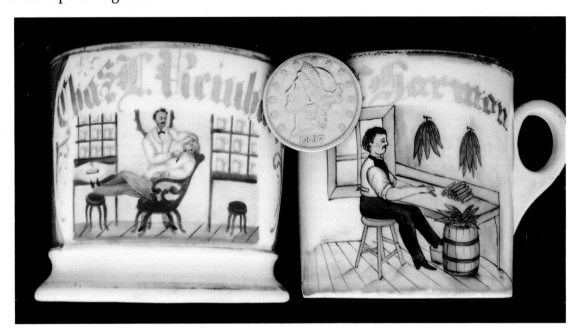

A gold coin next to the earlier, dull finish gold lettering.

A gold coin next to the later, mirror finish gold.

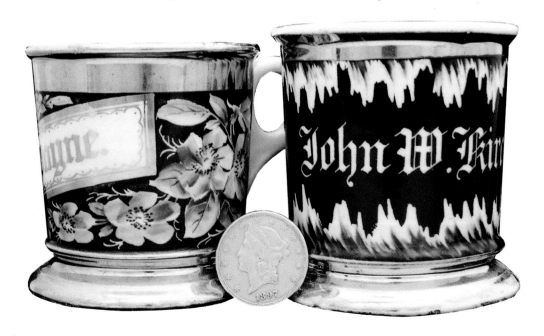

Here we see a tinsmith Occupational. The illustration is as good as the day it was sent to the original owner. But the gold has been completely worn off. If you roll the mug around under a light, you will usually find a shadow of the old gold work. This mug's original owner was named Harvey Miller.

Certain mugs will have this "gold shadow" under an illustration or another gold name. This is because the mug order had been canceled or returned. The barber supplier would remove the name and use the mug for another customer's order. Some collectors think that the placing of a new name indicates a fake, but in fact this was simple economy practiced by the supply house.

The Cartouch. These are the gold designs that flank the illustration. They can be very elaborate. Based on several examples over the years, I believe it is possible to tell where in the country the mug was decorated.

Mugs that I can trace from the Northeast have a sweeping fern type decoration, with a central design that is graduated, rather reminding one of ladder rungs. Midwest and western mugs have a grape vine type with three central curls. In both cases there are variations, but they are similar to the main examples. These elaborate designs are from the golden age. The early short blank mugs seldom have anything except an encircling wreath of leaves. From 1914 on, some mugs have a simple straight edge decoration.

Some large distributors, such as Koken of St. Louis had small sub-distributors in other parts of the country. So a number of mugs with midwest cartouches may be found in the Northeast.

The "straight-edged" cartouch.

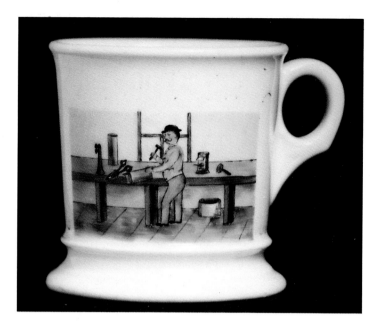

The tinsmith Occupational shaving mug.

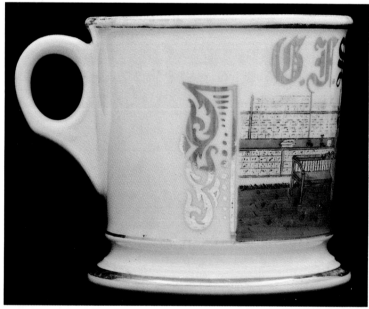

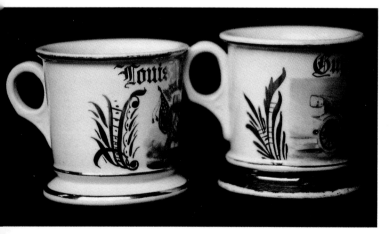

A cartouch from a mug decorated in the northeast, with a fern-like foliage and a graduated central design.

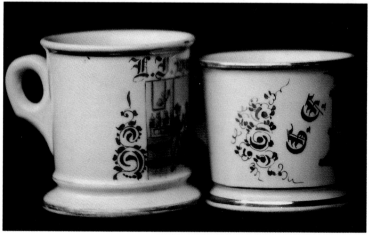

A midwest or western cartouch with a grapevine motif.

Barber Suppliers and China Decorators

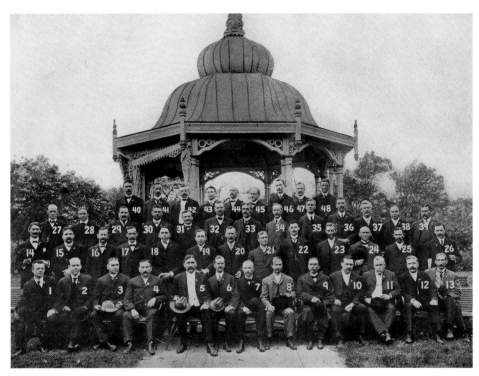

This 1904 photo is of the Midwest barber suppliers. Many of these men had large mug decorating departments, employing several decorators. From the number of men in this photo you can get an idea of how big a business this was.

There are several suppliers in this photo who have their stamp on the bottom of mugs. The more numerous examples you will find are: #5, Kern; #8, Koken; #9, Berninghaus; #20, Melechior.

The small object next to the mug, is a porcelain tobacco pipe bowl. This beautiful, highly decorated item is an example of fine German porcelain artistry. This illustration shows several views of a German army officer of 1888. Compare this to the mug, you can see the artistic similarity. The pipe bowl would have been difficult to decorate because of its small size.

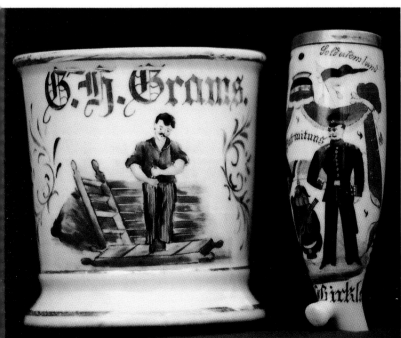

China decorators were hired to paint illustrations, not to follow their own whims. Almost every illustration was a copy from a standard catalog design. A plate or outline paper was impressed on the mug and the artist would finish the picture freehand. There were some requests that had to be painted totally by freehand. These mugs are referred to as "one of a kind".

Very few artists would sign their name. I would say that 95% of all mugs existing today aren't signed. An exception to this is J.R. Voldan of Cleveland. His mugs have a round stamp which states,"Decorated by J.R. Voldan". Mr. Voldan worked for the distributor Herold Brothers for a while. Sometimes mugs will have both his stamp and their's on the bottom. Phil Eisemann of Lancaster, Pennsylvania also signed his mugs.

There were china decorators who worked independently of barber suppliers, or worked for them on a contract basis. These men may have worked directly for the barber, being able to produce mugs cheaper and giving the barber a greater profit.

Having a decorator's name on the bottom of a mug adds some value. In past years collectors would feel confident about a mug's authenticity if it had a stamp, because fakes have no markings. Today I would suspect that a counterfeit stamp could be used to deceive collectors. However, I have never found a fake with a distributor or artist's stamp.

Here are some examples of supplier's marks found on the bottom of mugs.

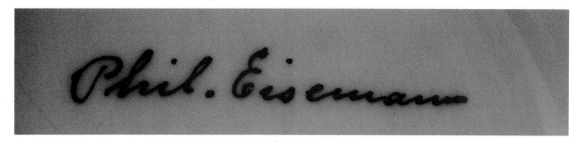

The signature of Philip Eisemann of Lancaster, Pennsylvania, as it appears on a mug of his design.

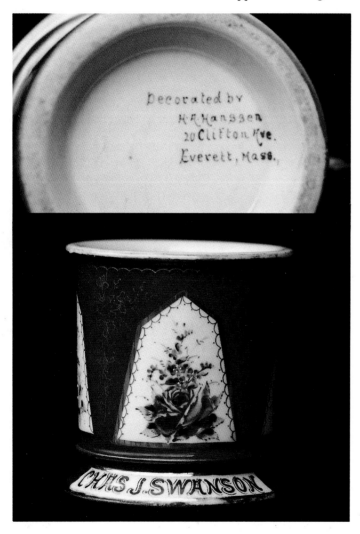

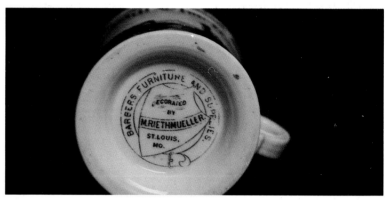

Mark for Barber's Furniture and Supplies, St. Louis, decorated by M. Riethmueller.

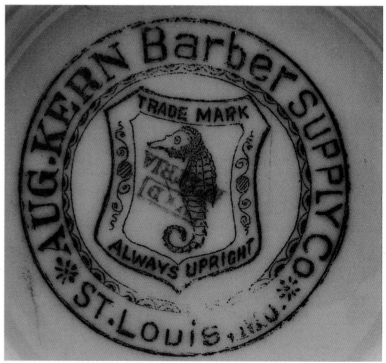

This beautiful Floral mug is an example of an independent decorator. The bottom of the mug has his name and address. "Decorated by H.A. Hanssen, 20 Cliffton Ave., Everett, Mass." I have tried to obtain some information about him. The Everett town records have a Hans A. Hanssen, listing his occupation as a China decorator. They show a son Harold born on February 7, 1907. After 1910 there are no further records. I have never seen another example of his work in any other collection.

A mark for Aug. Kern Barber Supply Co., St. Louis. The green stamp tells that the mug was manufactured in Austria.

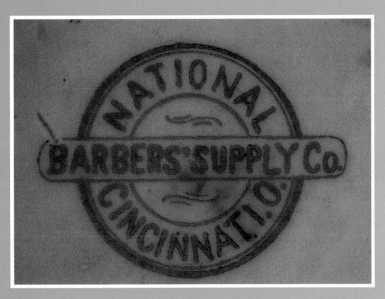

National Barber's Supply Co., Cincinnati, Ohio, stamp.

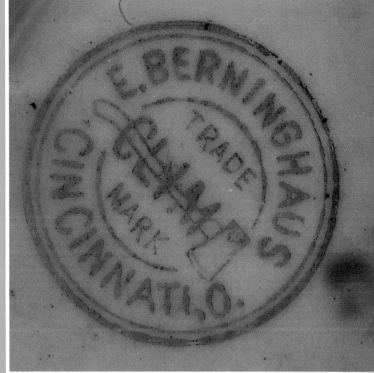

E. Berninghaus stamp with the "Clim-axe" trademark. Cincinnati, Ohio.

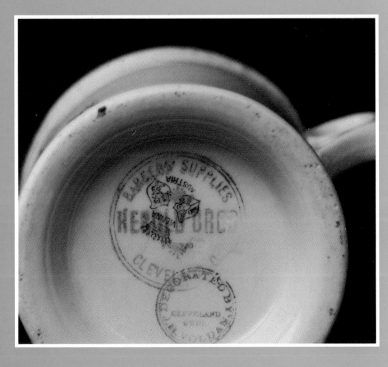

Here is a mug with everything. The green country of origin mark indicates the mug was made in Vienna, Austria. The large orange stamp is that of the Herold Brothers suppliers of Cleveland, Ohio. The small orange stamp is J.R. Voldan's, who was the decorator.

Chapter 2
Categories

There are five categories of personalized mugs. I have tried to rank their availability today, based on my collecting and dealing experience. In the categories of mugs certain determining factors can make a mug more difficult to find. I have used three grades to describe desirability and rarity: entry grade—easy to find; collection grade—average; advanced grade—difficult to find.

1. Gold Name: 30%
2. Floral: 20%
3. Decorative: 25%
4. Fraternal: 15%
5. Occupational: 10%

Gold Name

Gold Name mugs are the most numerous. One reason is they were the cheapest personalized mugs. They also began the mug era and ended it. In viewing old barber shop photos, I find that Gold Name and Floral mugs dominate the racks. This enlargement of a photograph of an old barbershop shows only one Occupational mug situated among many Gold Names and Florals.

I once interviewed a centenarian, Mr. James Grote of Chester, Connecticut, who owned a Gold Name mug that he bought in 1912. In our conversation I asked him why he didn't get a trade design (Occupational). His reply was, "I just wanted my name, nothin' fancy."

This may have been the reason that many rural shops had few Occupationals. People born in this country may have considered "fancy" mugs a waste of money. In most small towns everyone knew each other, and what they did for a living. An Occupational would have been unnecessary.

There is only one grade for Gold Name, gold initials, and monogram mugs: the entry grade. When collecting Gold Name mugs only acquire the best possible examples. The price range should be $20 to $40.

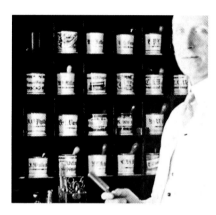

The mug racks of a 1912 barbershop. The whole image can be seen on the back cover of this book.

Mugs with Numbers

Not all shaving mugs were personalized. These numbered mugs were used in many barber shops to serve its transient customers. Some hotel and large train station shops had mugs numbered to over 100. The numbers can be in gold or black. In the barber shop photograph you can see a section of the barber's rack full of numbered mugs. These mugs are entry grade and are priced in the $20 to $30 range.

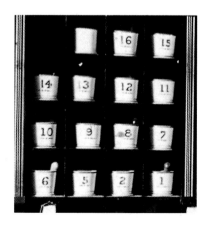

Numbered mugs in a 1912 barber shop.

Florals

Good Florals were as expensive as Occupationals to the original owners. Many china decorators were trained in the art of floral decoration in Europe. They may have spent their journeymen years decorating fine china exclusively with floral decorations. Some of the artistry of Floral mugs is exquisite.

The Floral category has both an entry and collection grade. A small Floral design which seems to flank or encircle the owner's gold name should be considered an entry grade mug. The high Floral design is the central graphic of the mug, usually a large example of a rose, a lily, or a bouquet. The second type is the more desirable and is collection grade.

Florals are common and you should be selective when collecting them, passing on mugs with any flaws. Some mugs, like the lily pad, in perfect condition can command prices in the $100 range. Most Florals range between $20 and $50. Like Gold Name mugs they satisfied those who wished a personalized mug, but didn't want to be associated with any trade.

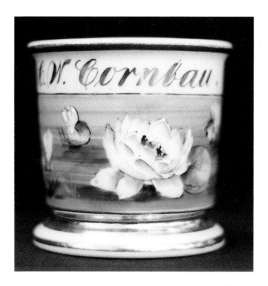

A water lily is the central feature of the this collection grade Floral.

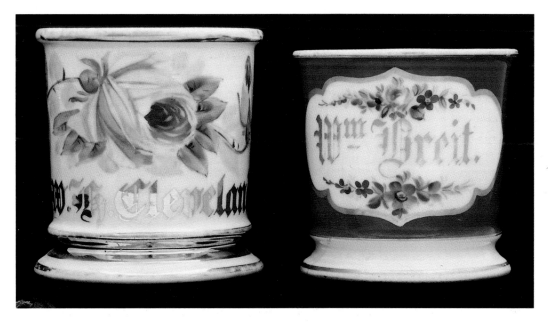

The collection grade mug, with the dominant floral graphic is on the left. On the right is an entry grade mug with flowers flanking the name.

Decoratives

Basically, any personalized mug not in the other four categories is a Decorative. Because of the many different types and prices, some attention must be placed here. With the exception of reproductions or fakes, this is where you can make a serious collecting mistake. Many mugs from this category are sold as the more valuable Occupationals.

Because of the large variety and types of mugs, this category is broken into several small subcategories. As with the other categories, there are three grades of Decoratives: entry grade, collection grade and advanced grade.

Entry Grade Decoratives

These are mugs decorated with abstract or geometric designs. They represent nothing in particular and fall into the same price category as Gold Name and basic Florals.

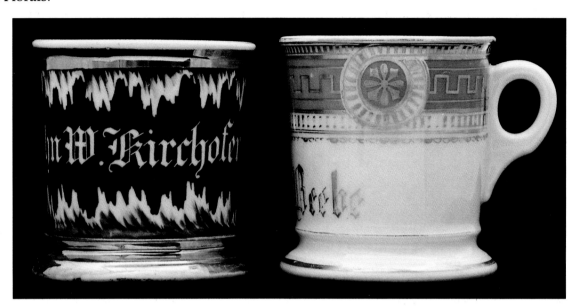

Typical entry grade Decoratives. Left: abstract frost pattern; right: geometric decoration.

Collection Grade Decoratives

Comic design. These mugs show animals involved in human activity. The most common examples are frogs, rabbits and monkeys. Some of these mugs aren't personalized, but they exist in the supplier's catalog, so they are considered of personalized quality.

Sometimes the comic design exploited racist humor. The common example is known as "The Razor Fight." It isn't personalized, but carries the same slogan as the previous example, "A Close Shave."

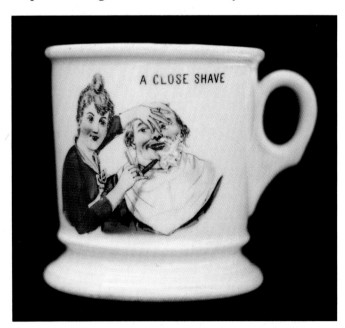

A comic design Decorative mug features a pretty girl giving a man a shave and the slogan, "A close shave."

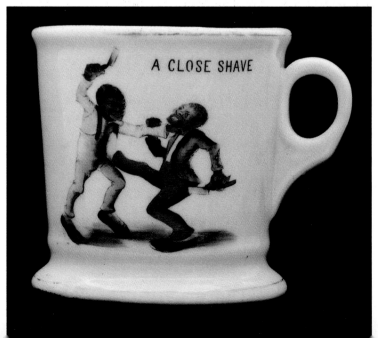

"Moon and Owl." This is said to have belonged to a night owl, someone who worked at night. So it is often assumed to be a night watchman's mug. It could also have belonged to someone who stayed in a saloon all night. Never buy a mug on an assumption.

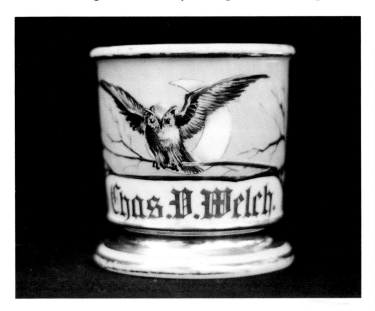

The "Moon and Owl" mug.

Pretty girl mugs. These are decal mugs which had been touched up by the china decorator. The use of decals is not a deterrent to collectors. They are also used on another mug called,"The Roman Soldier." Both of these mugs are personalized. I will cover non-personalized decal mugs in another section of the book.

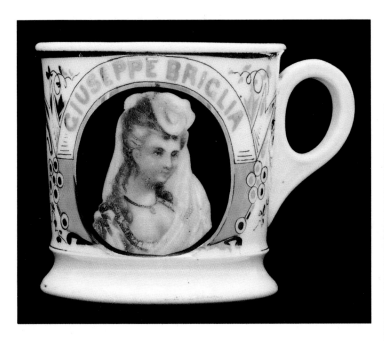

A typical "pretty girl" mug.

Child mugs. These have illustrations showing young girls and children in various scenes.

Scenic. Some examples of these are a pastoral farm view, a lake with a house in the distance, a sail boat on a lake and a snow or winter scene. The scenes are usually in a fancy frame or a circle and most of the subjects appear in miniature.

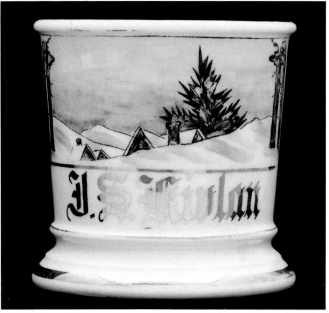

A wintry scenic Decorative.

The drape mug. Of all Decorative shaving mugs, these are most often misrepresented. Collectors have bought this mug believing it's an Occupational for an undertaker, an interior decorator, an actor, or theater owner. It is a drape mug and nothing else. It is common and several varieties exist. The price range should be from $50 to $90. If you have bought this mug and paid more, you're not alone.

A typical drape mug.

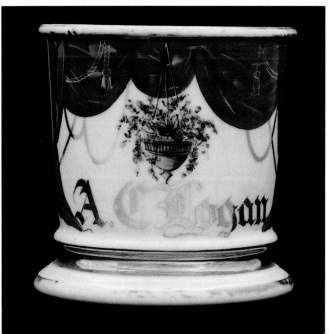

Bluebirds and Butterflies. There are several variations of these mugs. Some examples are detailed correctly, while others have fantastic colors, which existed only in the artist's mind. These are popular mugs, but only mugs with large illustrations should be acquired. Mugs with small birds around the lettering, and others showing a bird on a nest are common.

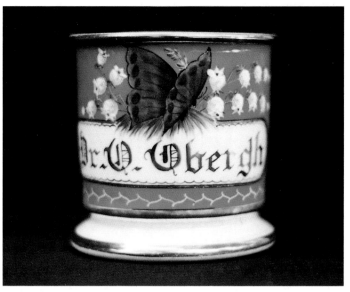

A nicely done butterfly mug.

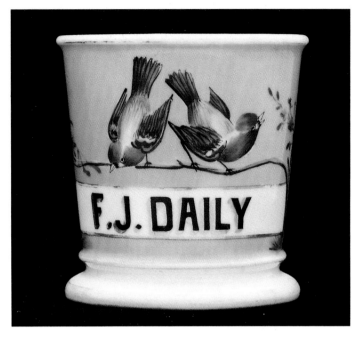

A bluebird mug.

Horse Heads. This is another common design with several variations. When a mug has a horse's head it is considered a Decorative, when it has a full body illustration, in most cases, it is considered an Occupational.

Horse head mugs are erroneously sold as blacksmiths or livery stables. If, in fact, the original owner were a blacksmith it still would not increase the mug's value, because it is not a true Occupational design.

A mug with two horse heads and two blue birds is said to represent a fraternal organization called "The Order of Chosen Friends." In old catalogues I have found this design in the Decorative section. It is a common mug and there is a similar modern reproduction.

On the left is an original "Order of Chosen Friends" mug, with a reproduction on the right.

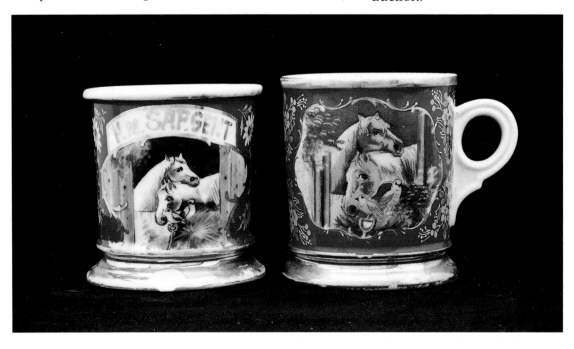

Hunt Decoratives. Illustrations of hunting dog's heads with game birds are considered Decorative, as is a dog encircled by a hunting horn.

Patriotic and nationalistic mugs These are sometimes referred to as eagle, flag, and shield mugs, and of the three the eagle mug is the most desirable. One common example is the eagle perched on top of the world with crossed flags. Sometimes one flag will be of another country, the owner's former homeland. There are many mugs with crossed flags only. The most common flags on the mugs are those of Italy, Germany and Ireland.

The shield mug is also common. It has great eye appeal and is popular.

The highest priced mugs in this category are the Irish Nationals. These mugs may in fact represent the "Ancient Order of Hibernians." This was a secret organization, and finding a mug with the A.O.H. emblem is difficult. Irish National mugs serve the same purpose of identification, without revealing membership in the A.O.H.

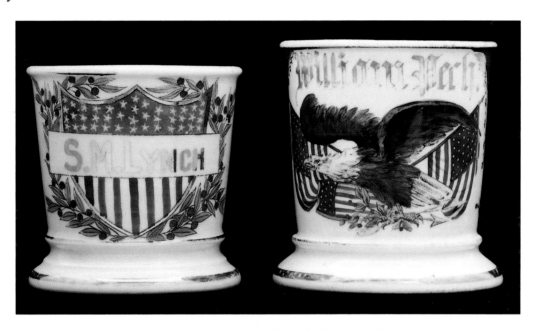

Two patriotic mugs. On the left is a shield mug and on the right is an eagle mug.

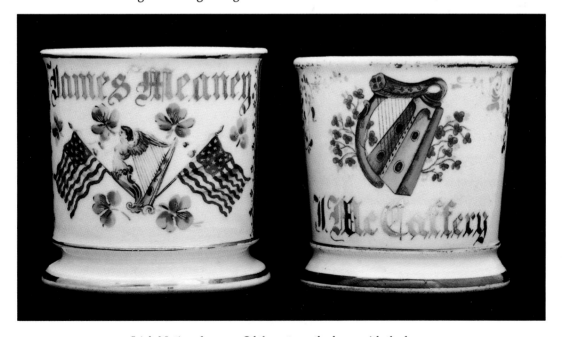

Irish National mugs. Of these two, the harp with the bare-breasted angel is the most desirable.

Advanced Grade Decoratives

The advanced grade Decorative is often confused with an Occupational. This is because the designs were originally chosen for their similarities to the Occupational designs.

Let's go back a hundred years. You are in your favorite barber shop and you are going to order a mug. Your favorite pastime is fishing, and you want a picture of a largemouth bass on your mug. As you go through the catalog you come across a mug decorated with an underwater scene with catfish. At this point you decide you want this mug instead.

So what's the difference? On seventy-five out of a hundred mugs, an advanced grade Decorative mug has the name running in a banner. On ninety out of a hundred Occupational mugs the name will be above or below the illustration.

To a new collector this may seem a trivial fact, especially since some advanced grade Decoratives can be as expensive as some Occupationals. But experienced collectors always want Occupationals. Sometimes a new collector can be fooled by a mug with a lot of flash. He may overpay because he thinks he is buying an Occupational.

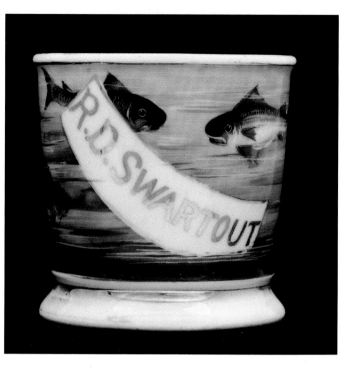

A high, advanced grade Decorative mug with the name running in a banner.

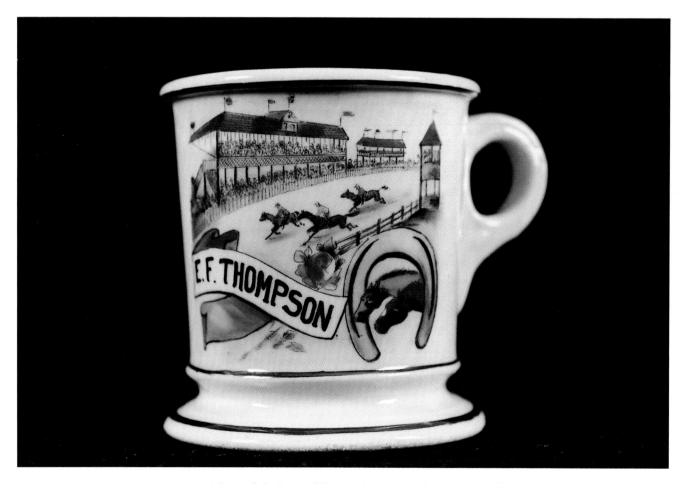

A beautiful advanced Decorative mug with a race track design.

Advanced Decorative mugs with race track scenes are often mistaken for jockey mugs. One such mug shows three horses in front of a full view of the grandstand, and there are two horse heads in a horseshoe at the end of the name. This is a beautiful mug and is worth $300-400. But, if it is thought to be an Occupational mug, it sometimes sells for more. Another Decorative mug shows a large illustration of a jockey watching a miniature racing scene.

Other types of Decoratives include one with a minstrel man beating a drum with the owner's name on it and one with a minstrel man sitting on a crescent moon with a banjo. A mug often sold as a newspaperman's Occupational shows two young girls, one black, one white, reading a newspaper.

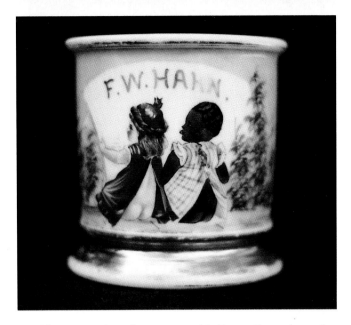

Two children reading the paper on this Decorative mug, make it possible that the mug will be mistaken for an Occupational.

The Grape Mug, Decorative or Occupational?

The mug with grapes could have belonged to a fruit dealer or a man who liked to eat grapes. The original owner is long gone so we don't know. But two facts exist so we can make a judgement: 1. The name is in a banner; 2. There is another scenic illustration on the mug.

We now know the name in a banner is a characteristic of a Decorative mug. The scenic Alpine view is a decorative illustration which is sometimes the sole graphic a mug. Because of these facts, this is classified as a Decorative. Let's say the mug had the same grape design, minus the Alpine scene and the banner name. If the name was across the base, or the grapes were altered so the name could be placed above, then I would call it a fruit dealer's Occupational.

Even if the original owner was a fruit dealer, the mug would still be considered a Decorative, because it has decorative characteristics.

And here is a grape mug which would be considered an Occupational. The original owner of either mug could have been a fruit dealer. But it is the characteristics of design that determines the mug's category.

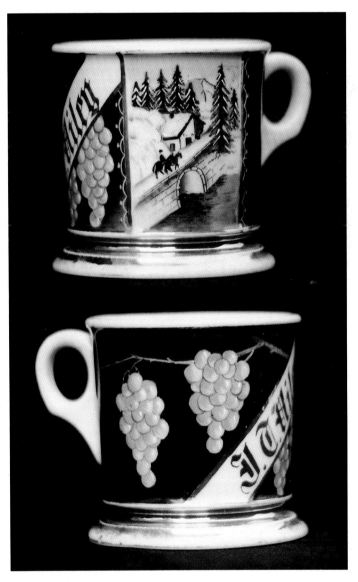

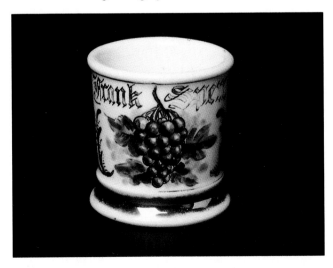

The grape mug with an alpine scene and the owners name in a banner. This is considered a Decorative.

Minor Categories

There are some mugs that fall into their own narrow categories. These mugs were all personally requested by the original owner.

Rebus. Sometimes an animal or object is used instead of a written description. The examples are "I am S. Woolton—who the 'devil' are you?" and Ben with a picture of a bear, the man's name was Ben Bear.

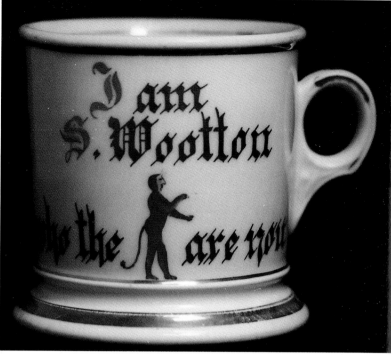

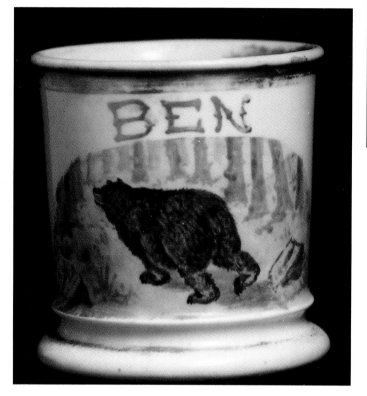

Rebus mugs.

Father and Son Mugs. Two mugs may have had the same design and belonged to a father and son or brothers. The Floral examples shown would be valued at $35 to $50 if they were sold separately. But because they are together they sell as a set and are worth between $150 to $200. Finding a set is difficult and they are desirable. They would be worth much more if Occupational.

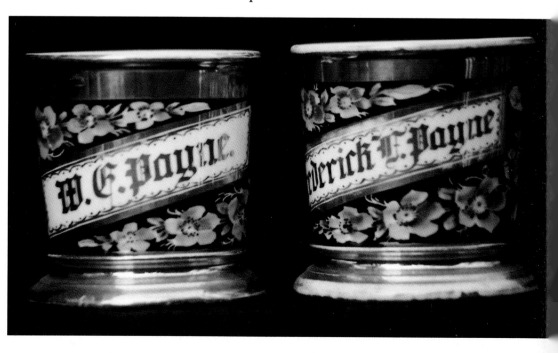

A father and son mug set.

Mugs with no name The peacock mug is a first class illustration, it also has a large amount of gold trim. It may be a Rebus mug, if the man's last name was Peacock. It may have been someone who owned or raised peacocks, and assumed everyone in town knew who he was. It also could have been a fancy "house" mug, that the barber would use on transient customers rather than a numbered mug.

I have seen other mugs without names, in each case the reason is a mystery. They were all on good blanks, with good artistry, gold trim and wraps. Everything you would want on a mug, except the owner's name.

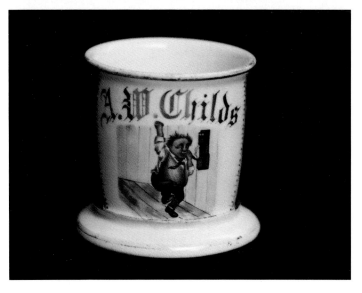

Our first example shows a man on a telephone in a rage, the present owner of this mug refers to it as "The Boss".

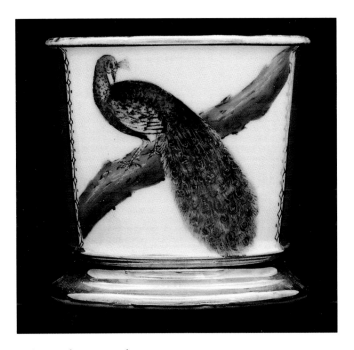

A nameless peacock mug.

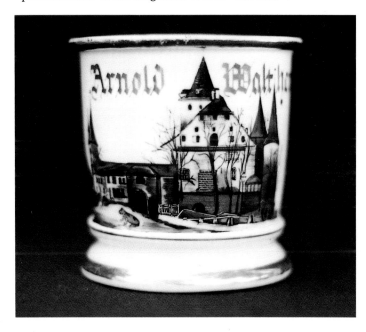

Here is a beautiful illustration of a castle, with a small frog in the road. Could this be a variation of an old fairy tale? Did the original owner wish for a kiss, so he could turn into a prince? Or was it someone who just liked castles and frogs? You be the judge.

Special Situations Some mugs have a specific illustration, but we aren't sure what the original owner had in mind. We can only assume the mug's meaning. Some of these could be comic characters from magazines or newspapers.

Here is a dog on top of his house frightened of geese. This would be a comic mug, except this is not a standard catalog design.

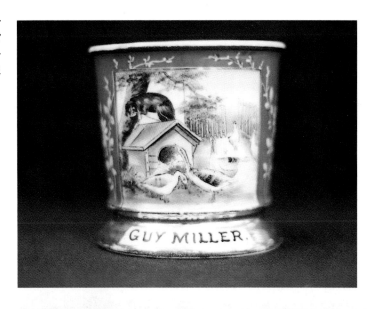

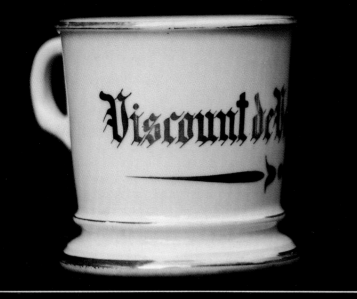

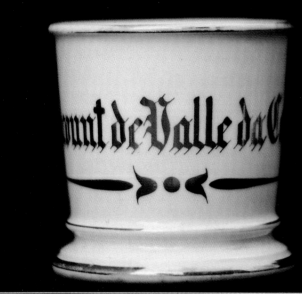

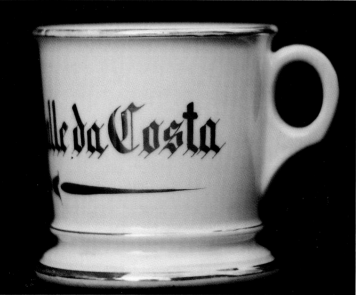

Occupational by courtesy. These are Gold Name mugs that have the occupation, profession, or title of its owner spelled out, rather than illustrated. These are technically Occupational mugs, but because of the lack of artistry they have a much lower value.

The examples show the mug of the "Viscount de Valle da Costa." Some documentation that came with the mug indicates that the owner was from a landowning family in the Isle Flories, Portugal. It also states that this man had a connection with the White Star steamship line out of Boston. The "Titanic" was of the same line. Is this a real Viscount's mug? Or did it belong to someone who was a legend in his own mind. This mug is a great conversation piece, and certainly a one of a kind. I only wish it had a coat of arms or family crest.

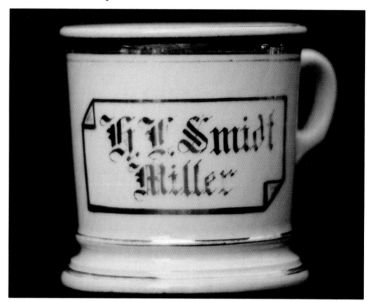

The miller Smidt's mug.

Mugs in Blue. Certain Decorative mugs are found with the entire graphics painted in blue. The most common example is the "Boy on a Tree Limb." The reason for this is unknown but the same illustration is printed in several old catalogs.

Because of its rarity I place a $125 to $150 value, on the Viscount mug. Standard mugs, such as Mr. Smidt's, the miller, are worth $50 to $75.

"Boy on a Tree Limb."

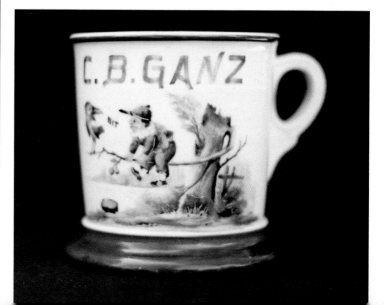

Awards and Presents Personalized mugs given as awards and presents are not common. Their status can make an advanced mug even more desirable. Two excellent examples are shown.

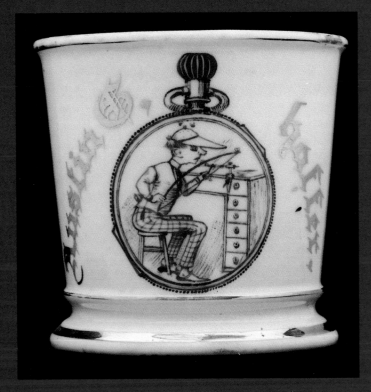

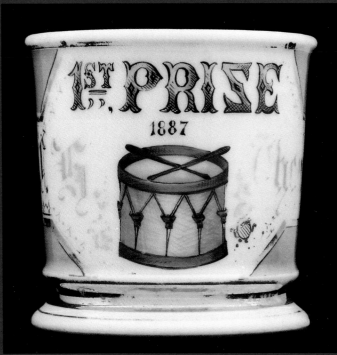

Here is an Occupational of a watchmaker. This has a very unusual design and the graphics are all in blue. This had to be a specific request. The use of blue in an Occupational is rare.

A prize for a drum competition. A drum mug is a desirable piece.

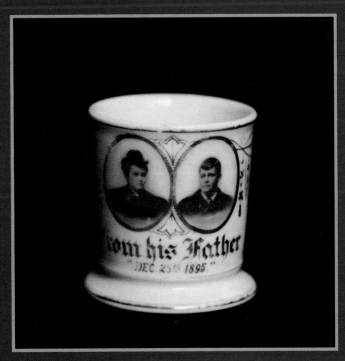

This is an extremely rare double photographic. This mug states "From His Father."

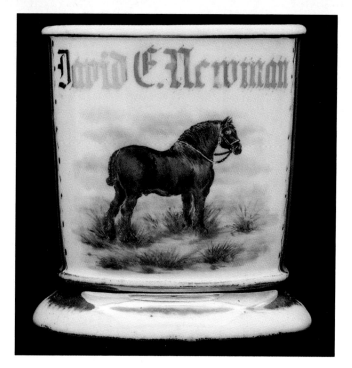

"A great big mug, with a great big illustration"

I have heard that quote from many experienced collectors. I don't always agree with this, but if all things are equal, the "big" example will usually be the most desired. The largest blank is 4 inches. The artist had a larger field to illustrate so he could enlarge the subject matter. Some suppliers charged more for larger mugs. This added price may have included or encouraged better artistry. The example shown is a four inch blank with a graphic of a Percheon horse. Here's the high quality artistry, almost photographic, that is the work of a skilled china decorator.

The original owner probably raised and sold draft horses. This mug had to have been a specific request, as the horse breed can be identified.

The Percheon horse Occupational.

Determining Factors

Before I discuss the Fraternal and Occupational categories, I have to explain certain artistic features which can increase or decrease the value of a mug. Fraternals and Occupationals are the most expensive and difficult to find. It is important to know how to distinguish between collection grade and advanced.

Additional Language

Additional descriptive wording can be in the form of gold script or black sign letters. It can be the owner's address or the manufacturer's name of some machinery or automobiles. On railroad mugs it identifies for which line the owner worked.

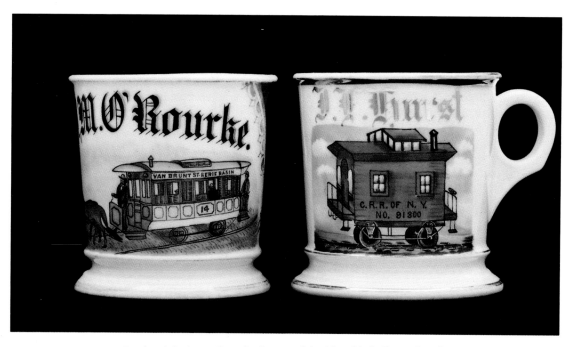

On the right is a railroad caboose of the New York Central with identification numbers, and, on the left, is a horse drawn trolley which shows the destination as"Van Brunt Street and Erie Basin." The car's number is,"14." Mr. O'Rourke was probably the only driver on that particular route.

"A better example than"

Sometimes a mug with a standard catalog illustration will have several additional items added to the graphics. These may have been requested by the owner, or an artist may have been inspired to add more to the mug than was necessary. The things to look for are peripheral subject matter.

In wagon and auto mugs there's a background subject known as "the industrial building." It can appear in the distance or close up, it can be a painted building or brick. It can be two or three stories, but it always has a flat roof. It may have been an addition when a customer requested a certain mug, but a "fancy" example.

Shown here is a standard horse and buggy mug, and a fancy example, with the industrial building in brick with an iron fence.

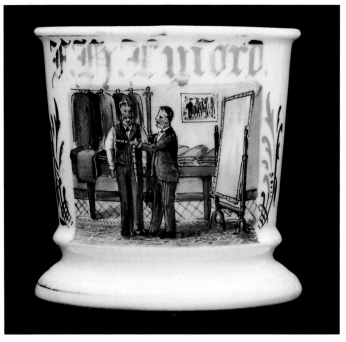

An Occupational of a men's clothing store. The standard graphics are the salesman with his measuring tape and the customer. The added features in this mug are the green rug, the racks of men's clothes, the full length mirror and, best of all, the advertising picture hanging on the wall.

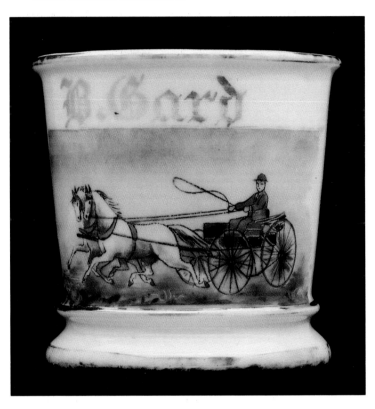

A standard horse and buggy Occupational.

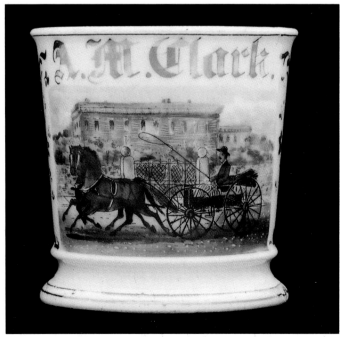

The horse and buggy with an industrial building and a iron fence.

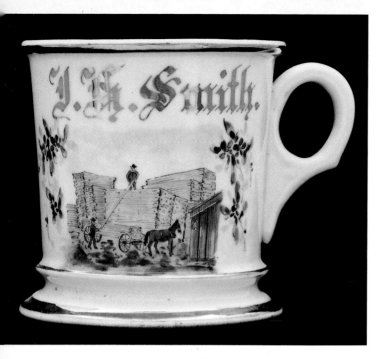

A lumberyard Occupational. This is the standard catalog design and a difficult mug to find. But the illustration is miniature, so the price will not be as much as the standard size illustration. However, it would be sought by collectors as an acceptable filler until they acquired a better example.

Miniature illustrations

This is the reverse of the "great big" mug theory. Some mugs have very small or miniature subject matter. It causes the collector to hold it close to tell what it is. This is considered a negative factor.

Positive Visual Impact

When looking at a collection of 30 or 40 mugs, one will catch your immediate attention. This may be due to superb artistry, facial details, or distinct graphics. It can be a combination of every positive determining factor previously mentioned. Sometimes this can raise the mug's price significantly. It is one feature that many advanced collectors look for.

A negative factor is incorrect artistic perspective, such as horses that are too small compared to a wagon or a man. Sloppy artistry is also a turn-off.

Fraternals

Occupationals and Fraternals go together like salt and pepper. Fraternals carry a lower price, but this could be an unrealized bargain. Fraternals are mugs that showed to which organizations the original owner belonged. All trade unions, patriotic organizations, religious organizations, and secret societies are classified as Fraternals.

The collector's goal is to acquire as many different types and hard to find examples as possible. Several Fraternal organizations have "degrees" or "levels." And they usually have separate emblems for each. It may be easy to find a Fraternal mug with a standard or entry level emblem. But it may be difficult to find the higher degrees of the same organization.

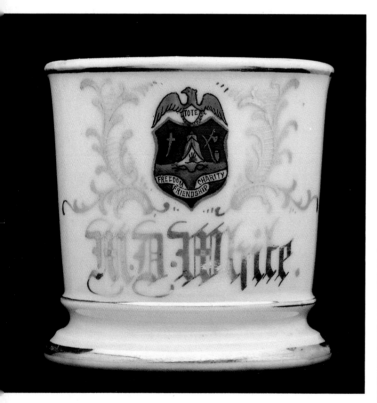

The more common shield design Redmen Fraternal.

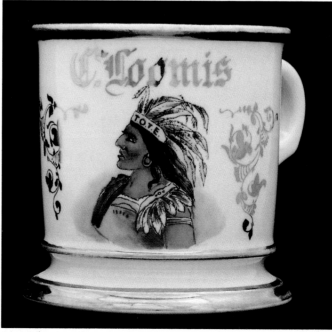

The "Chief" is a rare and popular Fraternal from the Independent Order of Redmen.

One example of this is the Independent Order of Redmen. It is a common mug with the shield design emblem. But the "Chief" is a rare and popular mug. The price difference is about $200. Redmen mugs have "T.O.T.E." on most examples.

You will see Occupational mugs with Fraternal emblems. These are referred to as "Occu-Frats". The value is determined by the rarity of both illustrations. An example of a low end mug would be a butcher's "steerhead," with an "Odd Fellow's" Fraternal emblem. A mug worth a premium would be a shoe store Occupational with an "Order of Owls" Fraternity. Both are desired and hard to find, so a collector could satisfy both collecting interests in one mug.

There are many Fraternals, with emblems that are unknown, some lasted only a few years and others were localized to one city. When these organizations died out no record was kept. But having one of these doesn't mean that you have a great and valuable mug. The mugs that are sought and valued by advanced collectors are the backbone of this category.

There are three grades of Fraternal mugs: entry grade, collection grade and advanced grade. Here are some examples.

Entry grade Masonic, Fraternal Order of Eagles, Odd fellows (Three rings), Jr. O.U.A.M. (American Mechanics), Knights of Pythias, Knights of Golden Eagle, Knights of Maccabee, B.P.O.E. (Elks), Order of Redmen (Shield), Ancient Order of United Workmen (A.O.U.W.).

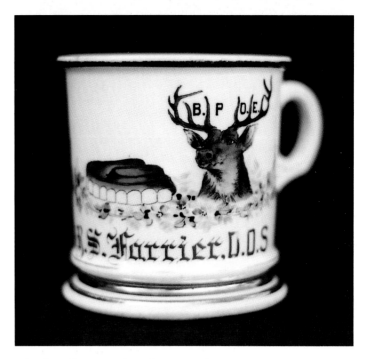

An Occu-Frat mug for a Dentist with a B.P.O.E. emblem. In this case the Occupational design is of greater value than the fraternal emblem.

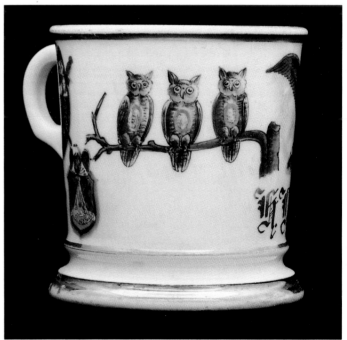

The six-emblemed Fraternal.

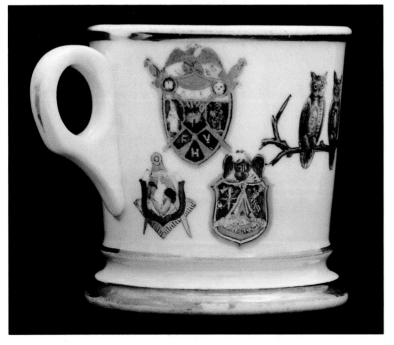

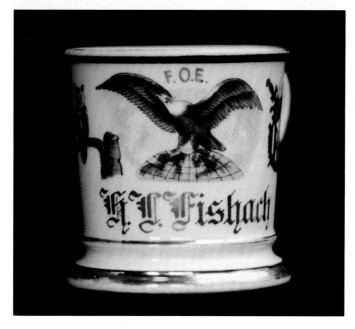

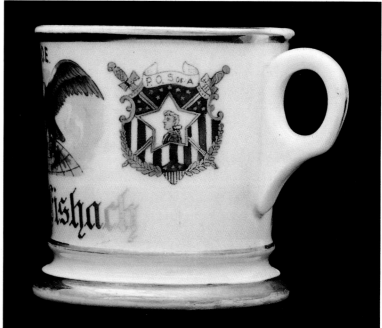

More of the six-emblemed fraternal.

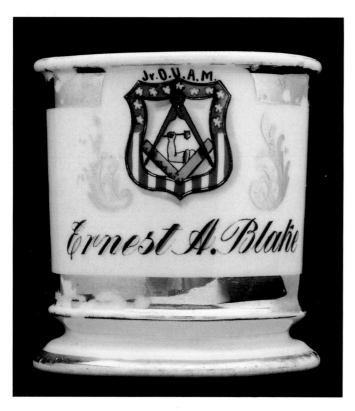

A basic, entry-level Jr. O.U.A.M. Fraternal.

Collection grade Grand Army of the Republic, Patriotic Order of the Sons of America, Woodmen of the world, Brotherhood of Railroad Trainmen, Sons of Veterans, Odd Fellows (Sword Over Bible with Eye), the Order of Moose, Knights of Columbus, Knight Templar (Cross and Crown), Brotherhood of Locomotive Engineers, Baker's Union.

Advanced grade Order of Owls, Ancient Order of Hibernians, American Legion, Order of Buffaloes, Knight Templar (in uniform), Ku Klux Klan, Redmen (Chief), Order of Independent Americans, Sons of Italy in America (Lion).

Multi-Emblems Multi-emblem mugs aren't unusual with two emblems. Sometimes mugs with three or four emblems can be found, but they are not common. A mug with five emblems is extremely difficult to find. I only know of two examples of a mug with six emblems. One of these is shown here and includes emblems for Knights of the Golden Eagle, Jr. O.U.A.M., Order of Redmen (Shield), Order of Owls, Fraternal Order of Eagles, Patriotic Order-Sons of America.

As with all personalized mugs, details are desired. Sometimes details and artistry can pull a mug into a higher grade even though the emblem is basically the same. The three mugs you see here are all Jr. O.U.A.M., but the determining factors dictate the price. The first mug shows the emblem in its most common form. This is an entry level piece. The second mug has two positive determining factors, flags that flank the emblem and a lodge number. The third mug has the same emblem but also has flags, open bible, and a little red school house, all of which are mentioned in the organization's charter.

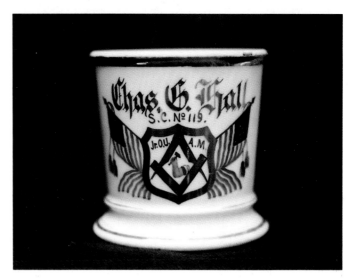

Another Jr. O.U.A.M. with flags and a lodge number.

Occupationals

Occupational shaving mugs are windows in time, allowing us to look back at a fifty year period of American history. They show us what work a man did and what tools he used. We see the items he made and products he sold, the animals he owned, the vehicles he drove, and the sports he played. It's folk art, it's Americana, and it's the most sought after article in barber shop collectibles.

There are two types of Occupationals, "working" examples and "symbolic" examples. Working examples show the man performing his work. Symbolic examples show tools, livestock, trains and retail products.

Certain mugs are classified as Occupationals, but actually represent a hobby or leisure activity. Mugs with sports figures, such as baseball players, generally did not belong to professional athletes. They were for people who played on local or factory athletic teams. A mug for a professional ball player would be worth much more. Mugs with hunting and fishing scenes are common and represent the largest recreational activity of its time.

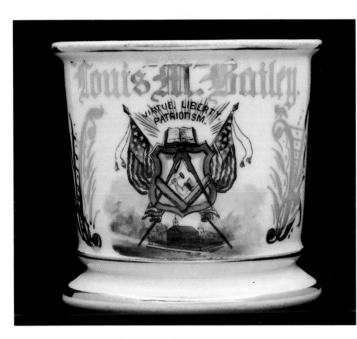

A Jr. O.U.A.M. with several factors that make it a most desirable piece.

Here are Occupationals showing a working cabinet maker and the symbolic block plane.

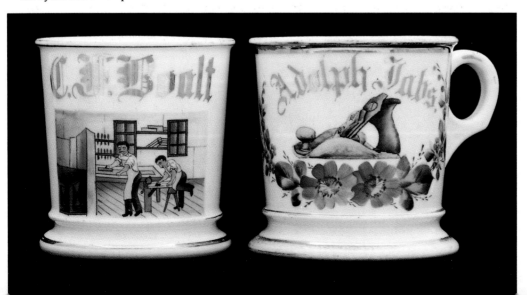

Musician mugs are from local marching bands, which were prominent at this time. A mug for a music teacher or band leader would be worth much more.

Like Fraternals, there are three grades of Occupationals: entry grade, collection grade, and advanced grade.

Entry Grade

The word "entry" is somewhat misleading. All Occupationals are difficult to find. But there are some which are found more often than others. The collectors call them the "three B's".

Butcher-Steerhead. Because every town had at least one butcher, this is the most common Occupational. As the design was popular many variations exist. Butcher's mugs with a sheep's or pig's head are more difficult to find.

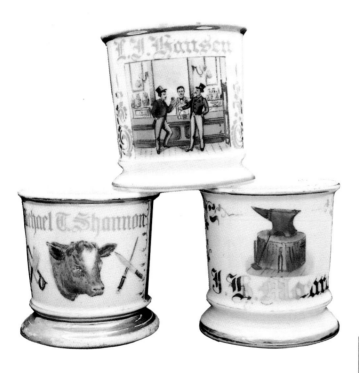

The "Three B's", Butcher, Bartender, and Blacksmith, are common entry grade Occupationals.

Bartender. Saloons were numerous at this time, so these are very common Occupationals. Alcoholism was rampant, which eventually led to prohibition. The standard illustration shows two customers with the bartender. Mugs with the bartender alone or with many customers are slightly more desirable.

Blacksmith. Another common occupation which would have existed in every town. The two standard examples of blacksmith Occupationals are an anvil with tools and the working blacksmith.

34

Several other mugs can be in the entry grade or collection grade depending on the degree of artistry and general overall appearance of the mug. These include a pharmacist's mug (mortar and pestle), a tinsmith's (lead furnace and soldering iron), a stationary engine, and a simple railroad locomotive. All of these could be considered collection grade if their artistry and determining factors were better than average. The entry grade consists of about 30% of all Occupational mugs.

Collection Grade

This grade represents the largest percent of Occupationals, about 60%. These mugs would have belonged to men in the average trades and occupations of the day. The price would be determined by the degree of artistry and the determining factors.

Advance Grade

Oscar Wilde once said,"I am very easy to please, I'm always satisfied with the best." The best, when speaking of shaving mugs are those with rare subject matter, and obtaining these is the main goal of all collectors. Rarity can be determined by graphics with one or more of these factors: "one-of-a-kind," professional and common labor, the unusual, or advanced machinery.

One-of-a-kind. Ask any old collector what his best mugs are and he will show you his "one-of-a-kind." These are mugs that have no standard illustration. There are two different types of these. The first is an artistic interpretation of a photograph or sketch. While the subject matter may not be rare, the non-standard illustration is. A good example of this is the "Tracy" mug. This artistry is a likeness of a

Tracy mug.

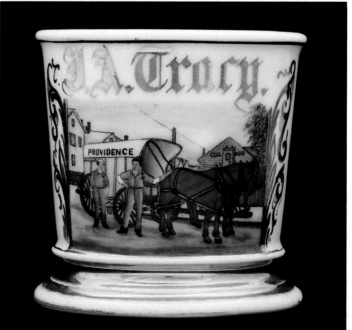

photograph. We can determine this by observing details which have nothing to do with the "Providence Wood and Coal Company". Notice the telephone pole in the background, the three family-style houses to the rear of the wagon. This is how the street really looked. Add to this the body language of the boss man and the helper behind him, the non-standard angle of the wagon and a building which indicates a wood and coal delivery business, and you have a unique image.

The second type is more truly a one-of-a-kind mug. It is the ethnic Mayor mug of James Donegan. Here we see a bearded man in a top hat and tails. He is holding the flag of his native land, Ireland. The base of the mug has additional wording, "Mayor Hewitt". I have never seen another mug similar to this. The subject matter is too abstract to have ever been included in a distributor's catalog. It might have been submitted as a sketch, but there is probably much artistic interpretation in the graphics.

Professional and Common Labor Professionals include doctors, dentists, lawyers, and professors. Only a few men of the shaving mug era went on to college, and, because of their small numbers, their mugs are also few. This category is also open to politicians and wealthy non-professionals, such as factory owners.

Their opposites, the common laborers, are also rarely portrayed on mugs. There were millions of these workers, but very few would have a mug showing them performing non-prestigious labor. A Gold Name, Floral or Decorative would have been selected instead. Common labor Occupationals would include boot blacks, street sweepers, and gandy dancers. Two examples of this type of mug are shown here: Mr. Gram's, who was a brick molder, and Mr. Hosly, who was a saw filer. These mugs represent people who were proud of their work, and were willing to spend a day's wages, to have it illustrated on their mug.

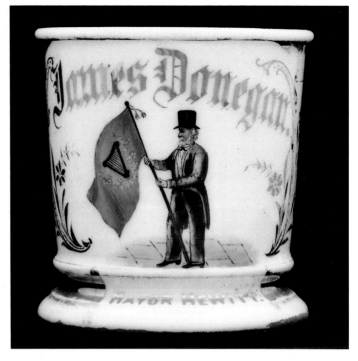

The Mayor mug.

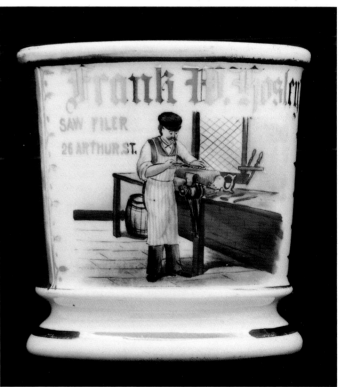

A saw filer's mug with his address. Perhaps this served as a subtle advertisement as it sat on the barber's shelf.

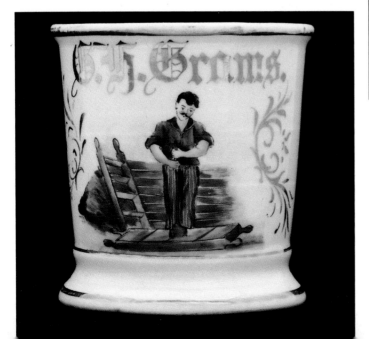

A common laborer's mug representing a brick molder.

35

The Unusual These were occupations or trades which didn't exist in every town. Mugs portraying these are rare, but not one of a kind. Two examples of these are an oil well worker, and a tugboat sailor.

Heavy Machinery Heavy machinery was not rare, but having it illustrated on a shaving mugs was. Some of these machines include steamrollers, tractors, and a piledrivers. Certain automobile and truck mugs which can be identified as rare manufacturers are also considered to be in this group. Shown here is a railroad steam shovel, known as a "wrecker".

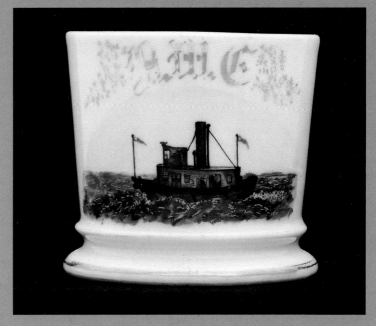

A tugboat sailors Occupational.

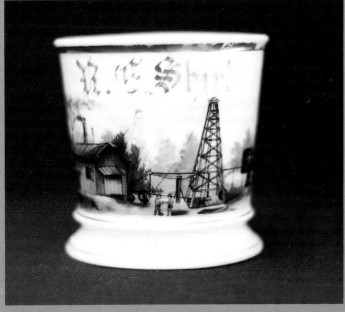

An unusual oil well worker's Occupational.

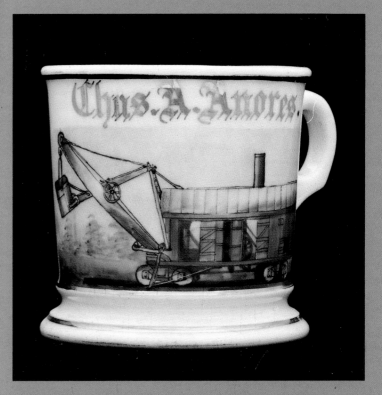

A railroad steam shovel.

Photographic Mugs

These are unusual and difficult to find. Some collectors desire this type more than any other. Others do not think they are folk art and don't care for them.

The original owner would submit a photograph to the barber's distributor. At the decorating department, they would take a photograph of the submitted picture, and with a special process print it right on the mug. It would then get a name and gold trim and be fired like any other mug.

There are two types of photographic mugs, portraits and working scenes.

Portrait These can be square or oval. They show the portrait of the owner but not necessarily his occupation. Sometimes they aren't personalized.

Working Scene Sometimes these are pictures of a factory interior, railroad locomotive, wagon, or a shop. Sometimes the artist would touch-up the finished product to make it more distinct, and add color.

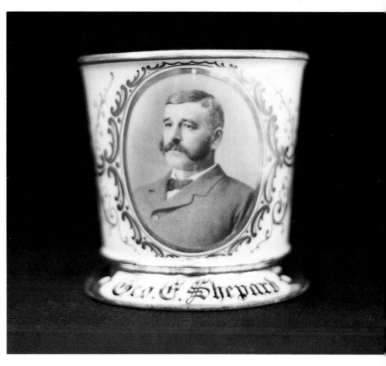

A portrait mug with George Shepard.

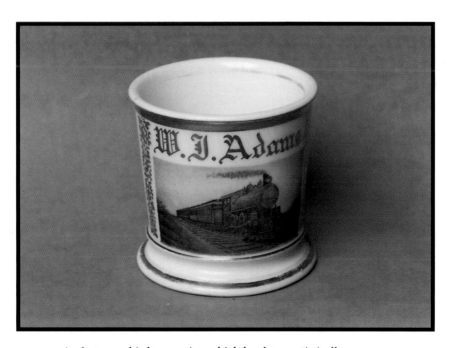

A photographic locomotive which has been artistically enhanced.

Mugs with Two Illustrations

All of these mugs are personal requests. In one way these are all "one of a kind," because no catalog ever advertised a dual illustration mug. But both graphics could be of a standard catalog design.

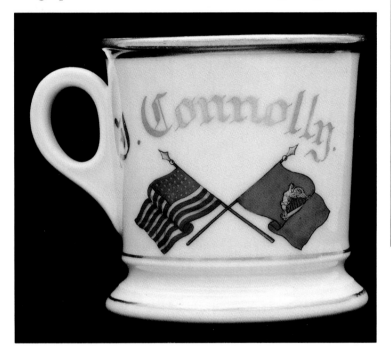

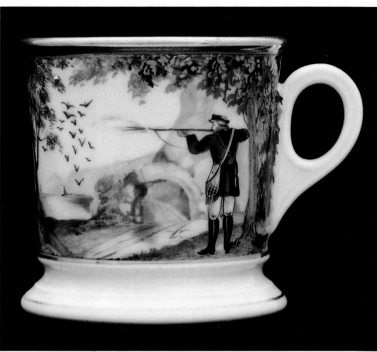

An example of a flag mug (Irish-American), with a Hudson River style hunting scene. The hunt scene is unusual, because the original owner asked for a fancy background.

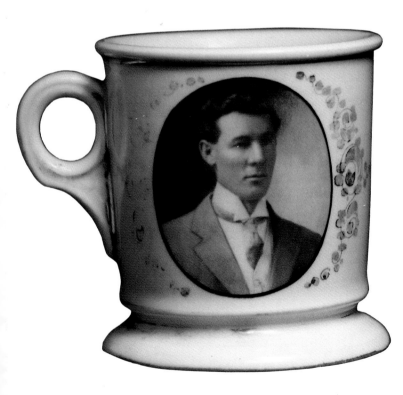

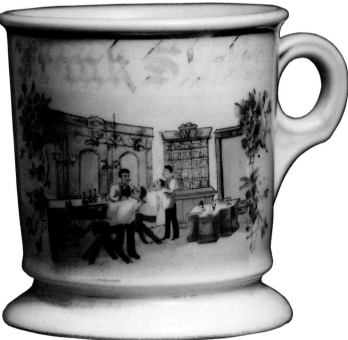

Here is a rare example of an occupational scene and a photographic. The photo is the owner of the barber shop. The painted illustration is a barber shop interior. This is a nice graphic, but a standard catalog design.

Chapter 3
Shaving Mugs

Barber Supplier's Catalogs

When a man became a steady customer at a particular shop, the barber would suggest that he should have his own mug. The barber would have a catalog illustrated with several examples of mugs. When a customer found an illustration he wanted, the barber would take his order and send it to his supplier. The finished product was identical to the catalog example, except the owner's name would be on the mug.

The supplier's price was fixed in the catalog. The barber could charge whatever retail price he wanted. A mug that cost the barber two dollars was probably sold for three dollars to the customer.

Catalogs are difficult to find, and range in price from $50-$200. Features you should look for when buying them are:
1. Good overall condition—no torn or missing pages and covers intact.
2. Mug era catalogs—newer catalogs without mug illustrations are undesirable.
3. Numerous mug illustrations.
4. Color illustrations

The following pages are examples from the Holzhauer catalog. Catalog pages 122 and 123 have prices for mugs which aren't illustrated. Page 122 lists decorated shaving mugs as "trade design" and "society emblems". Turn to pages 236 and 237 of this book for a the catalog list and prices. You will never see the words, "Occupational" and "Fraternal" in any old catalog. These are terms that are used by collectors.

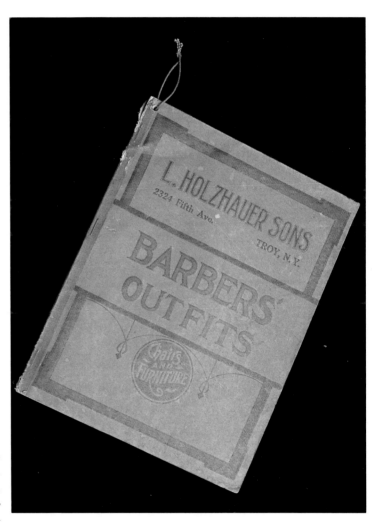

The catalog shown here is from L. Holzhauer Sons, Troy, New York. The string at the top of the catalog was for hanging on the barber shop wall.

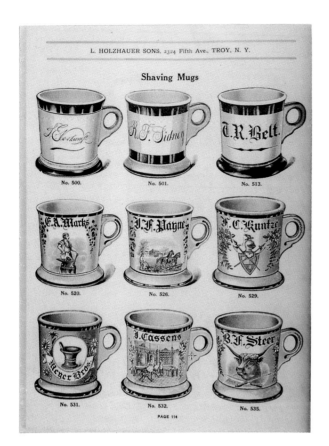

Shaving Mugs

No. 500. No. 501. No. 513.

No. 520. No. 526. No. 529.

No. 531. No. 532. No. 535.

PAGE 114

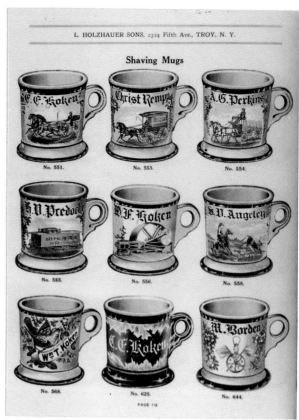

Shaving Mugs

No. 551. No. 553. No. 554.

No. 585. No. 556. No. 558.

No. 568. No. 625. No. 644.

PAGE 116

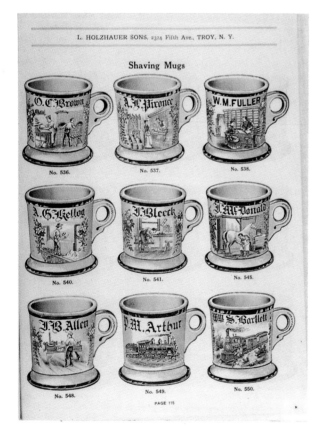

Shaving Mugs

No. 536. No. 537. No. 538.

No. 540. No. 541. No. 545.

No. 548. No. 549. No. 550.

PAGE 115

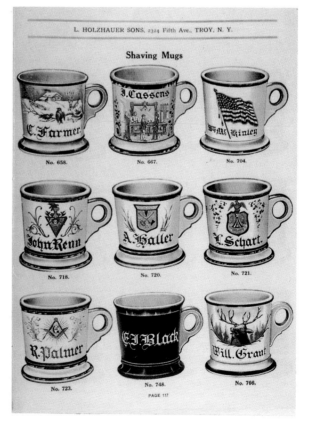

Shaving Mugs

No. 658. No. 667. No. 704.

No. 718. No. 720. No. 721.

No. 723. No. 748. No. 766.

PAGE 117

Shaving Mugs

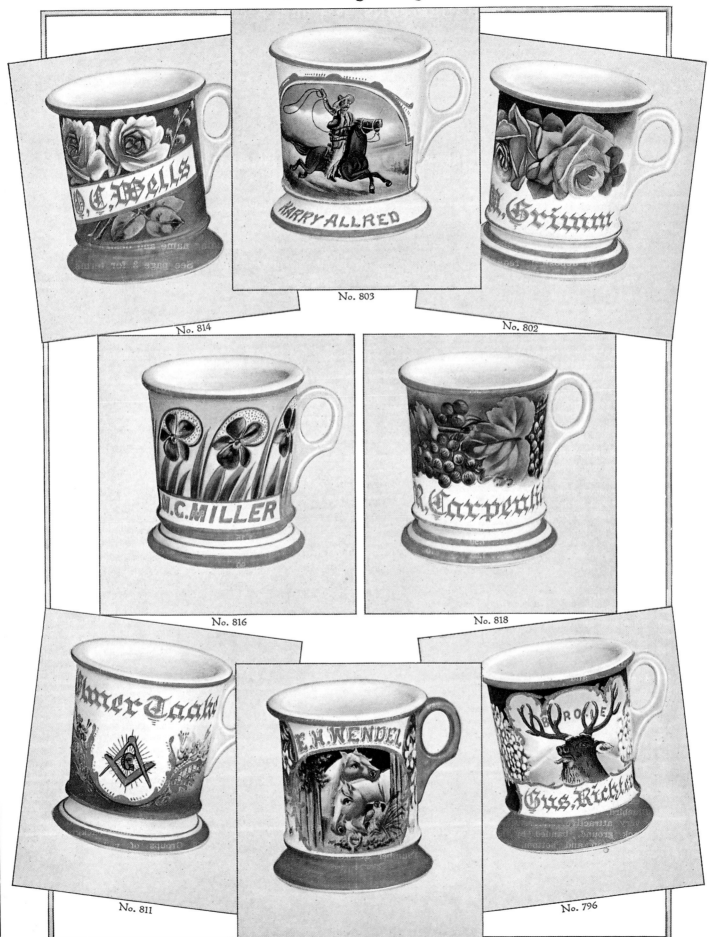

No. 803

No. 814

No. 802

No. 816

No. 818

No. 811

No. 799

No. 796

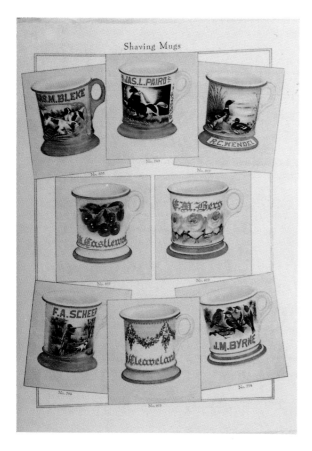

Mug Examples

Here are mugs from several collections. In critiquing them, I found it necessary to use my own experience and that of the present owners, to interpret the correct category and designation. Some mugs had documentation with them when they were acquired by their present owners. Mugs such as "the piano" example is captioned as a "Hartford band leader." You can't tell this by looking at the mug alone. The mug would be sold as a piano with "documentation." This may or may not increase the price. What would increase the price is "band leader, Hartford CT.", as additional wording in the graphics.

Gold Name

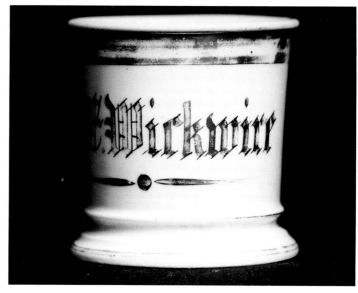

Gold Name. *Courtesy of Mrs. Fred Willman.*

Gold Name, fancy. *Courtesy of Morris Pickerell, Jr.*

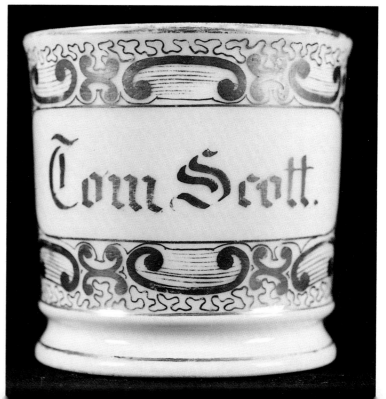

42

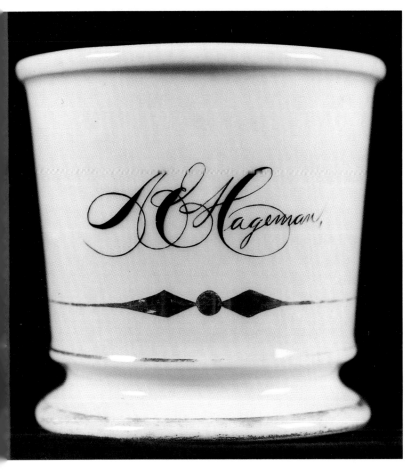

Signature facsimile. *Courtesy of Morris Pickerell, Jr.*

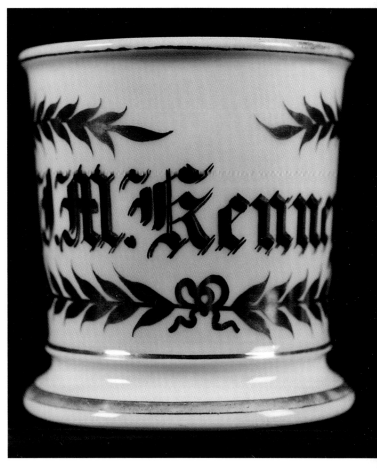

Black name with gold. *Courtesy of Morris Pickerell, Jr.*

Floral

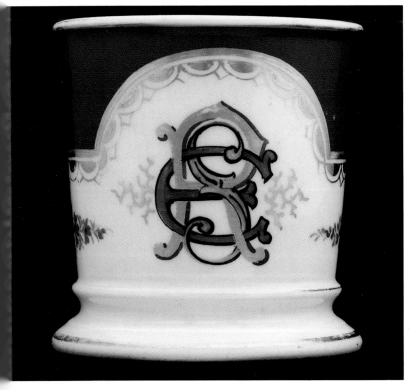

Monogram. *Courtesy of Anthony Gugliotti.*

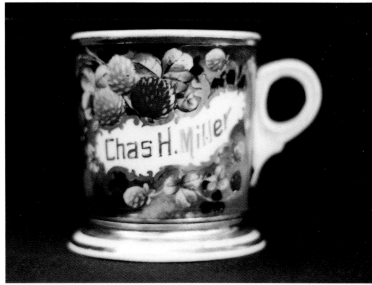

Thisel. *Courtesy of Dr. Ralph Nix.*

43

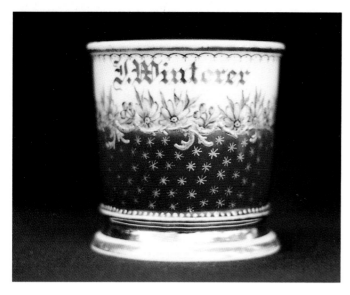

Yellow Flower, red fabric decoration. *Courtesy of Dr. Ralph Nix.*

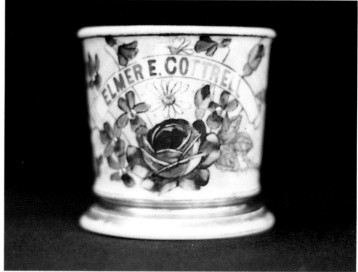

Rose and Violets. *Courtesy of Dr. Ralph Nix.*

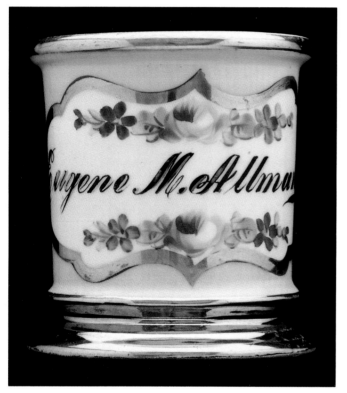

Small design, yellow wrap. *Courtesy of Dr. Ralph Nix.*

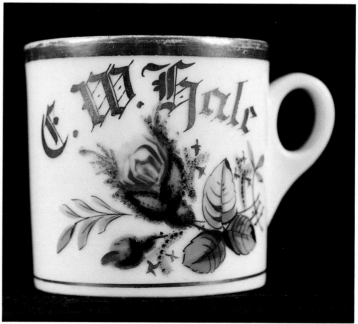

Rose. *Courtesy of Morris Pickerell, Jr.*

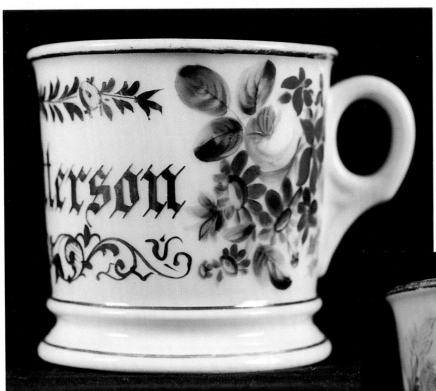

Side decoration, rose. *Courtesy of Morris Pickerell, Jr.*

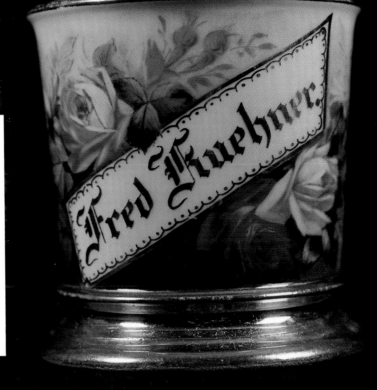

Roses. *Courtesy of Morris Pickerell, Jr.*

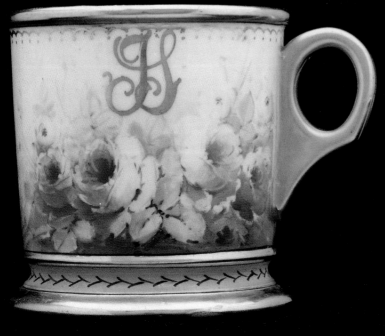

Monogram with roses, excellent artistry.
Courtesy of Anthony Gugliotti.

45

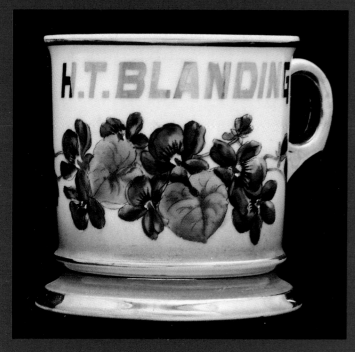

Violets. *Anonymous.*

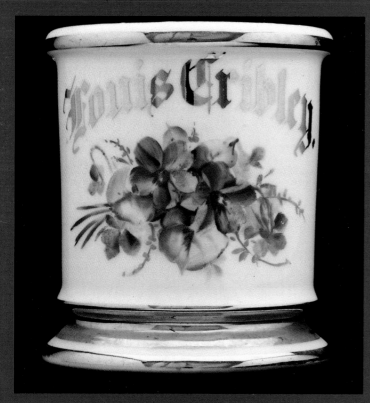

Violets. *Courtesy of Anthony Gugliotti.*

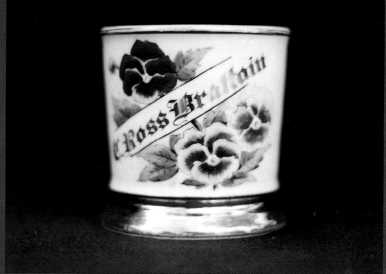

Pansy. *Courtesy of Dr. Ralph Nix.*

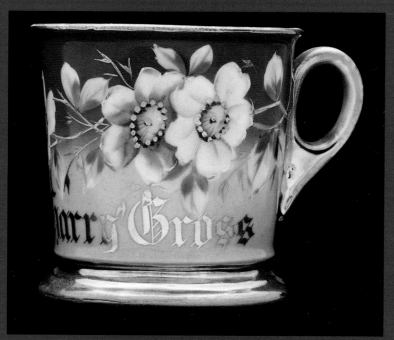

Morning Glory. *Anonymous.*

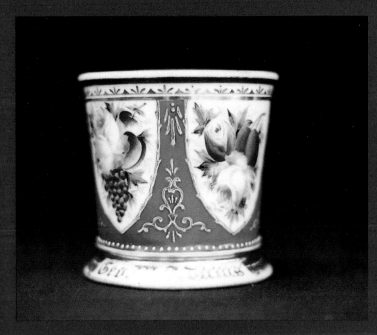

Floral with fruit. *Courtesy of Dr. Ralph Nix.*

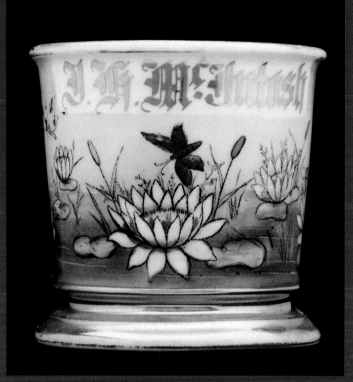

Lily pad. *Courtesy of Anthony Gugliotti.*

Decoratives

Scenic

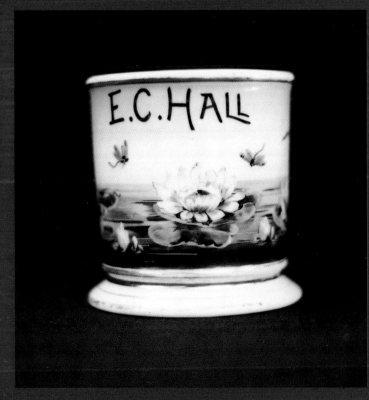

Lily pad. *Courtesy of Dr. Ralph Nix.*

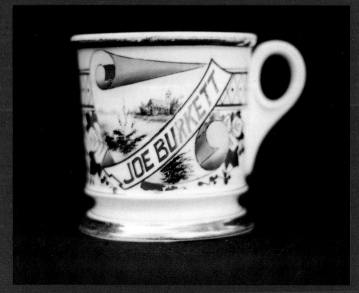

House within scroll. *Courtesy of Dr. Ralph Nix.*

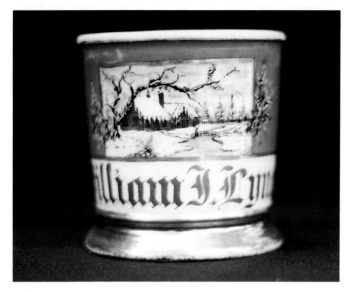

Snow scene. *Courtesy of Dr. Ralph Nix.*

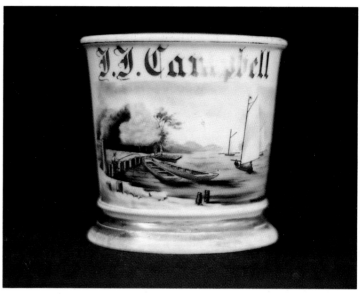

Lake scene, boats and a boy fishing. *Courtesy of Dr. Ralph Nix.*

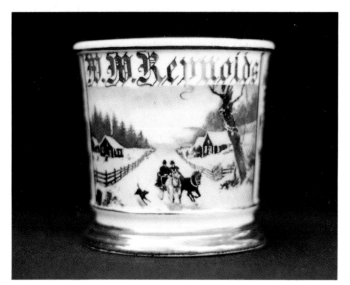

Winter scene, advanced. *Courtesy of Dr. Ralph Nix.*

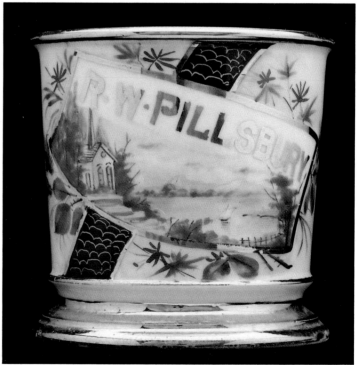

Lake scene with church. *Courtesy of Anthony Gugliotti.*

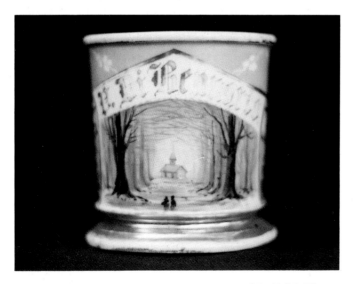

Winter scene, church through trees. *Courtesy of Dr. Ralph Nix.*

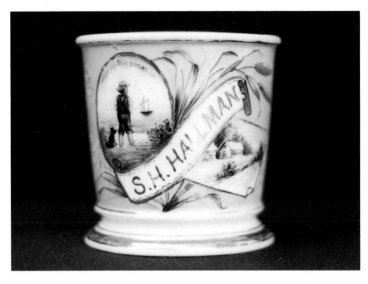

Double scene, boy and cabins. *Courtesy of Dr. Ralph Nix.*

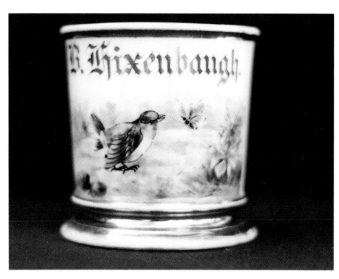

Butterfly and bird. *Courtesy of Dr. Ralph Nix.*

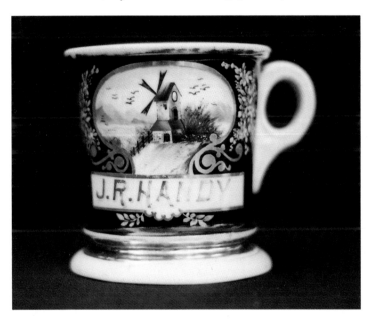

Windmill. *Courtesy of Dr. Ralph Nix.*

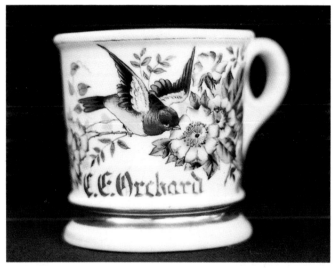

Bluebird and flower. *Courtesy of Dr. Ralph Nix.*

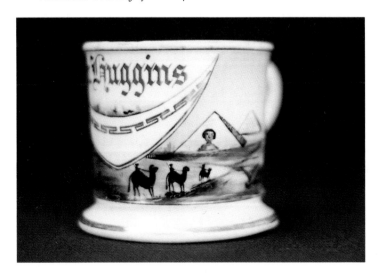

Sphinx and pyramids. *Courtesy of Dr. Ralph Nix.*

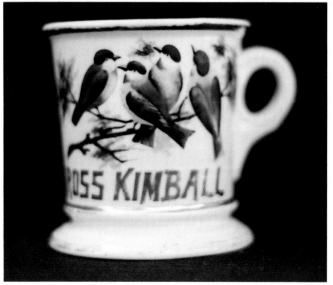

Four bluebirds. *Courtesy of Dr. Ralph Nix.*

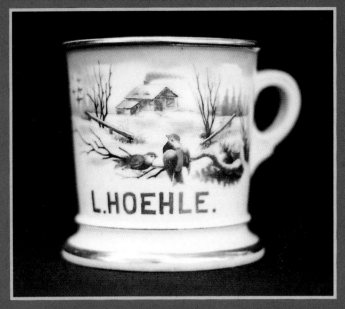

Birds, cabin in winter. *Courtesy of Dr. Ralph Nix.*

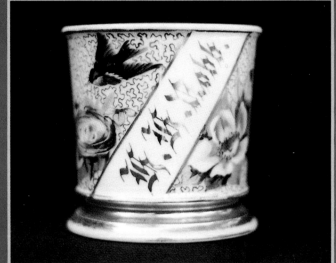

Bird with nest. *Courtesy of Dr. Ralph Nix.*

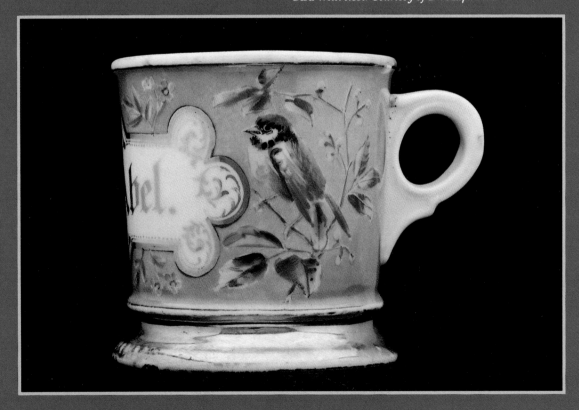

Bluebird, side illustrations. *Courtesy of Anthony Gugliotti.*

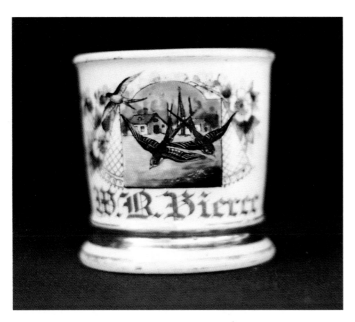

Birds and cabin scene. *Courtesy of Dr. Ralph Nix.*

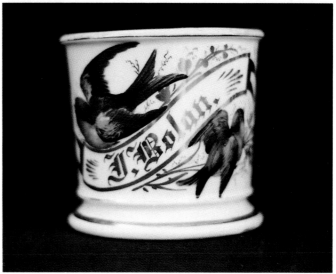

Two bluebirds. *Courtesy of Dr. Ralph Nix.*

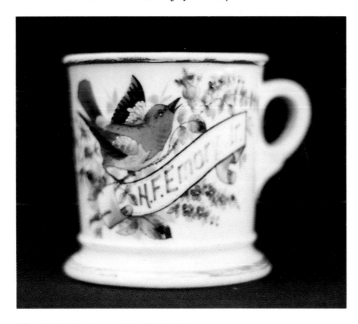

Bluebird. *Courtesy of Dr. Ralph Nix.*

Bluebird on branch with a butterfly. *Courtesy of Dr. Ralph Nix.*

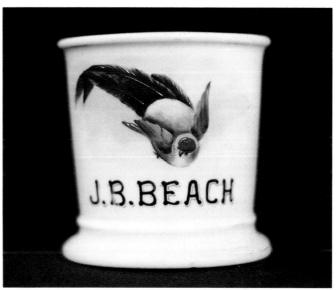

Bird of paradise. *Courtesy of Dr. Ralph Nix.*

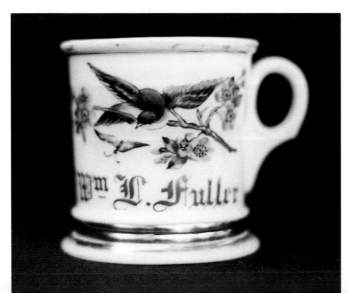

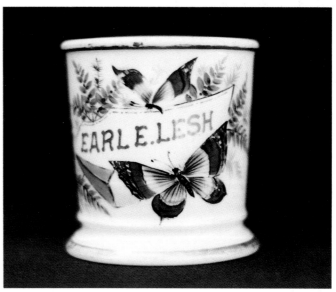

Butterflies. *Courtesy of Dr. Ralph Nix.*

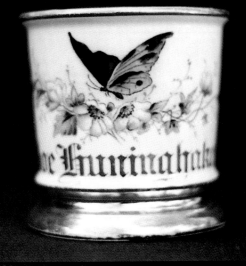

Butterfly and flowers. *Courtesy of Dr. Ralph Nix.*

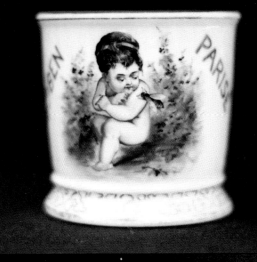

Baby with bee. *Courtesy of Dr. Ralph Nix.*

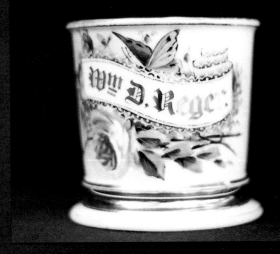

Butterfly and rose. *Courtesy of Dr. Ralph Nix.*

Girl Design

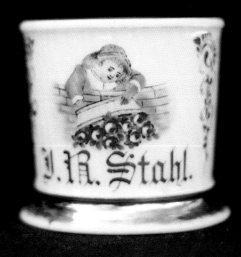

Girl dropping basket of flowers. *Courtesy of Dr. Ralph Nix.*

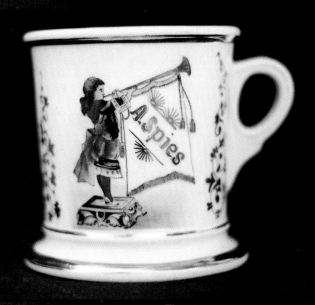

Girl with horn. *Courtesy of Dr. Ralph Nix.*

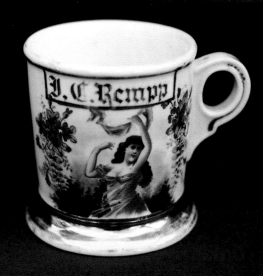

Dancing girl. *Courtesy of Bernard Lukco.*

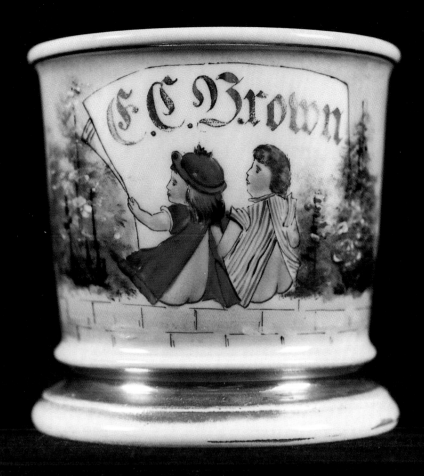

Girls reading a paper. *Courtesy of Morris Pickerell, Jr.*

Hunt Decoratives

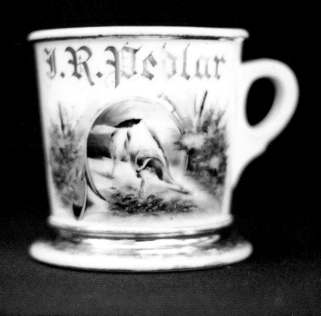

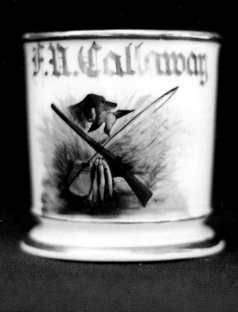

Dog inside of hunting horn. *Courtesy of Dr. Ralph Nix.*

Fishing and hunting gear with dog. *Courtesy of Dr. Ralph Nix.*

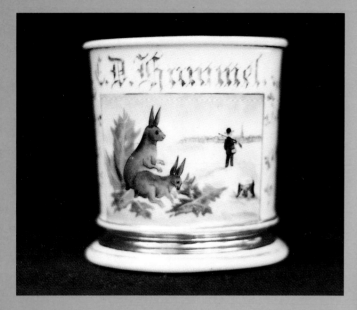

Rabbits watching hunter. *Courtesy of Dr. Ralph Nix.*

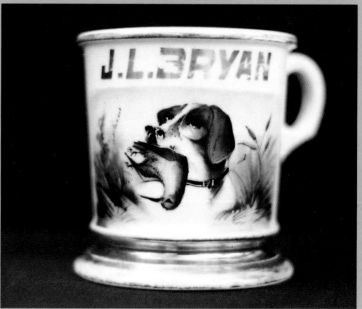

Dog's head with bird. *Courtesy of Dr. Ralph Nix.*

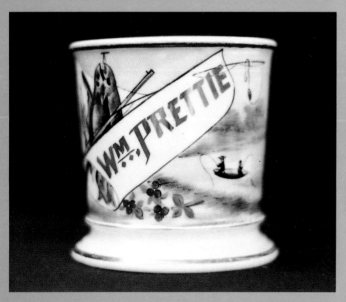

Fishing gear with catch. *Courtesy of Dr. Ralph Nix.*

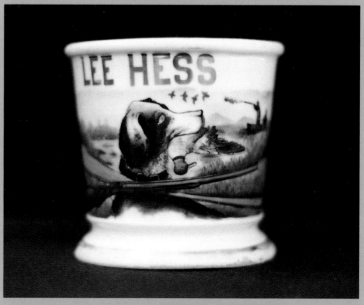

Dog's head with duck. *Courtesy of Dr. Ralph Nix.*

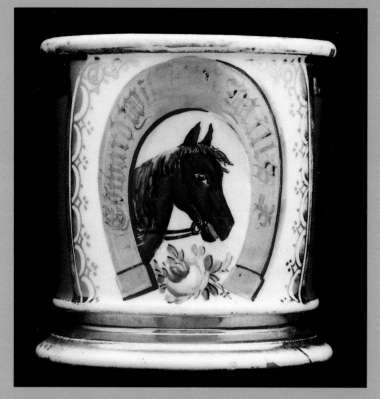

Name in horseshoe. *Courtesy of Anthony Gugliotti.*

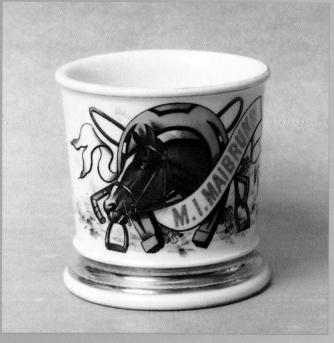

Horseshoe, whips and stirrups. *Courtesy of David Giese.*

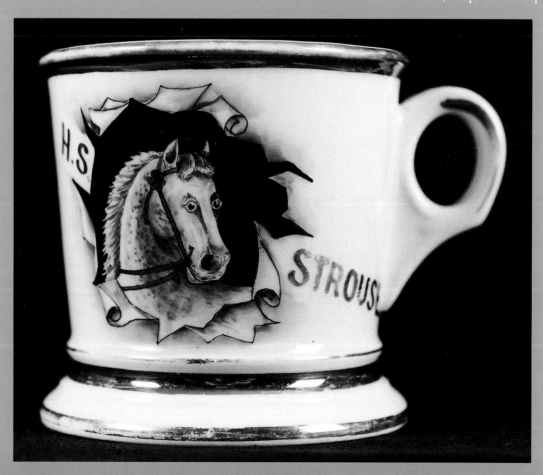

Horse head breaking through paper. *Courtesy of Morris Pickerell, Jr.*

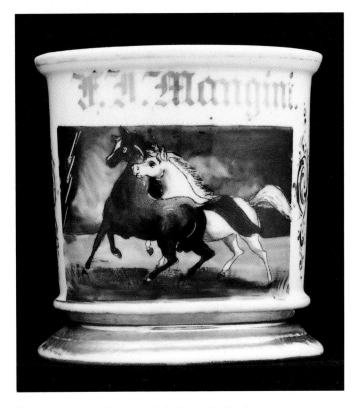

Horses in storm. *Courtesy of Anthony Gugliotti.*

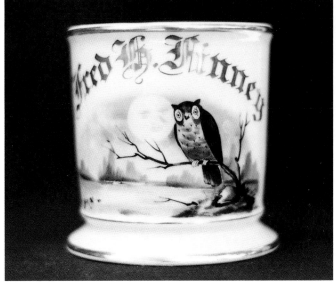

Owl and moon. *Courtesy of Dr. Ralph Nix.*

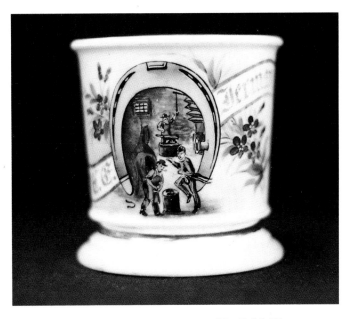

Humorous blacksmith scene. *Courtesy of Dr. Ralph Nix.*

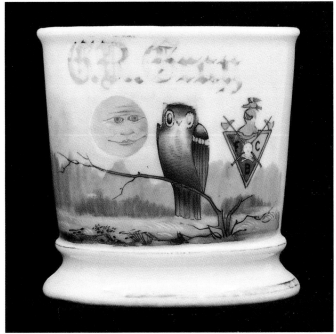

Owl and moon, K. of P. Fraternal. *Anonymous.*

Two owls. *Courtesy of Dr. Ralph Nix.*

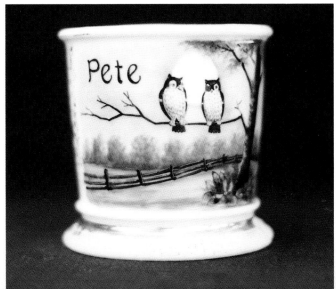

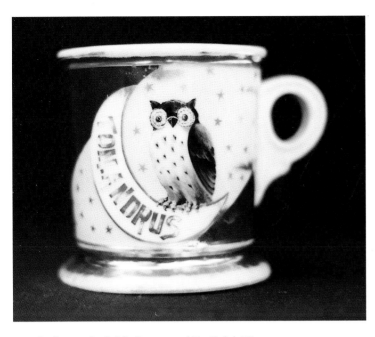

Owl, stars in field. *Courtesy of Dr. Ralph Nix.*

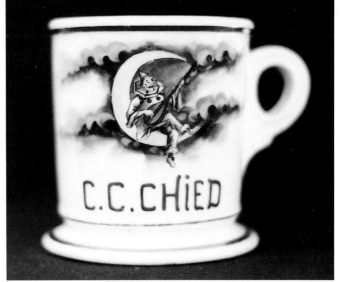

Minstrel, clown on moon. *Courtesy of Dr. Ralph Nix.*

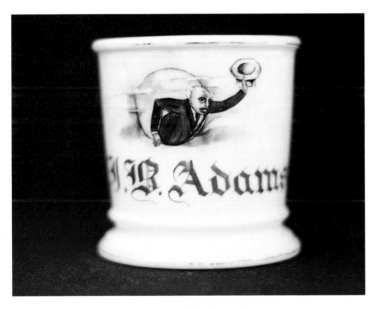

Man in the moon. *Courtesy of Dr. Ralph Nix.*

Moon. *Courtesy of Dr. Ralph Nix.*

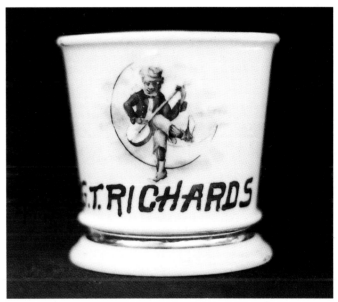

Minstrel, man on moon. *Courtesy of Dr. Ralph Nix.*

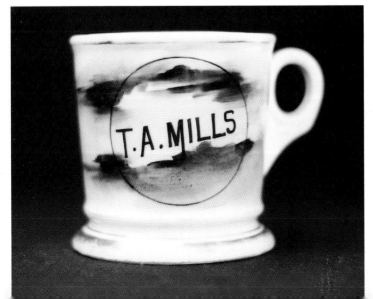

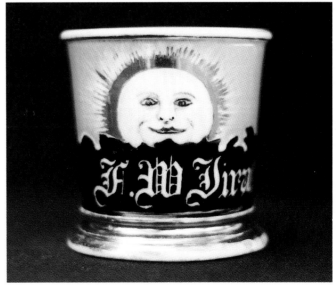

Sun. *Courtesy of Dr. Ralph Nix.*

Frogs

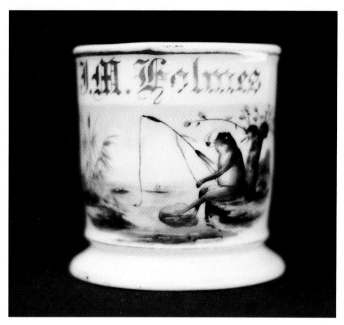

Frog fishing and smoking a pipe. *Courtesy of Dr. Ralph Nix.*

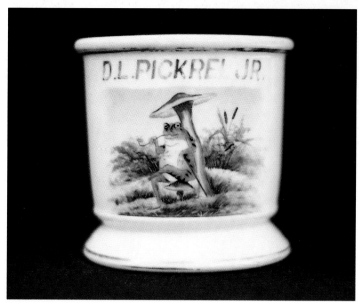

Frog under mushroom, smoking. *Courtesy of Dr. Ralph Nix.*

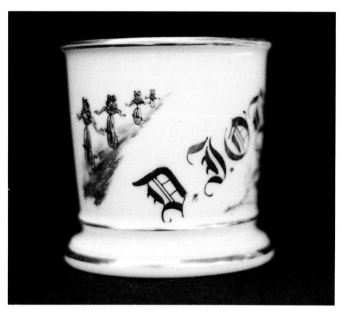

Frogs on bicycles. *Courtesy of Dr. Ralph Nix.*

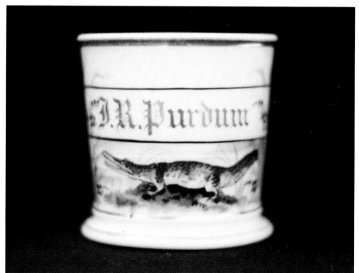

Alligator. *Courtesy of Dr. Ralph Nix.*

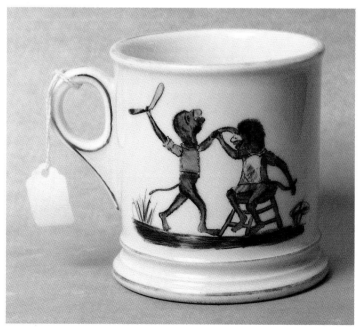

Monkeys, shaving scene. *Courtesy of David Giese.*

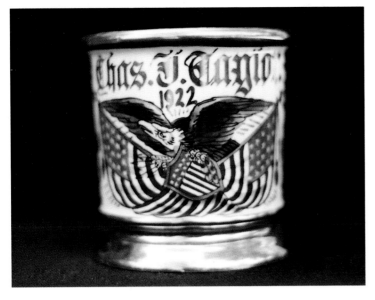

Eagle, crossed flags with shield. *Courtesy of Dr. Ralph Nix.*

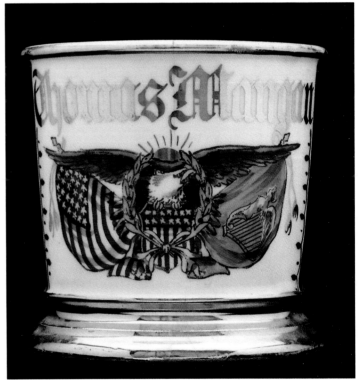

Eagle, lightning bolts, black wrap. *Courtesy of Dr. Ralph Nix.*

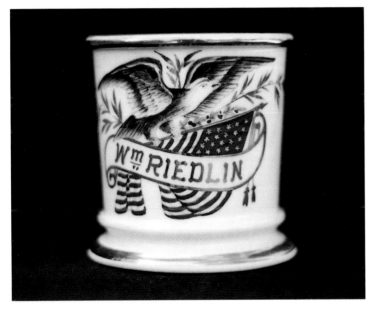

Eagle with flags. *Courtesy of Dr. Ralph Nix.*

Irish American. *Courtesy of Anthony Gugliotti.*

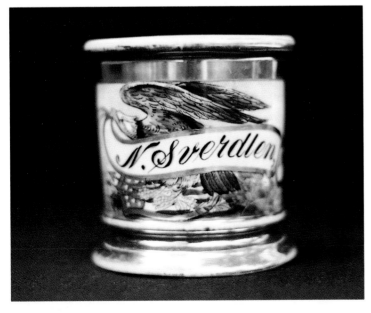

Eagle, shield with banner in beak. *Courtesy of Dr. Ralph Nix.*

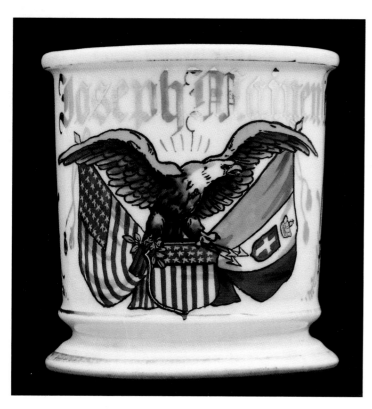

Italian American. *Courtesy of Anthony Gugliotti.*

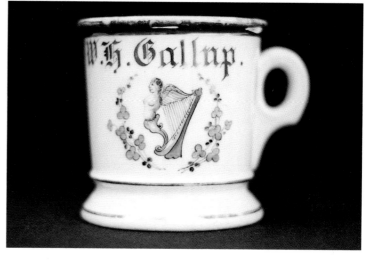

Irish national, harp with angle. *Courtesy of Dr. Ralph Nix.*

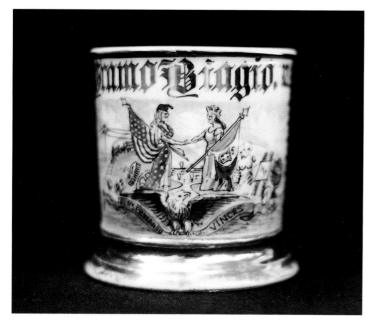

Italian American, Liberty and Columbia. *Courtesy of Dr. Ralph Nix.*

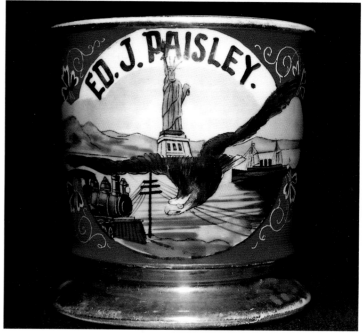

Land of opportunity and industry. *Courtesy of Raymond and Theresa Jones.*

Other Decoratives

Fan with roses. *Courtesy of Dr. Ralph Nix.*

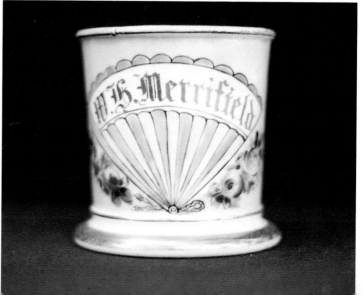

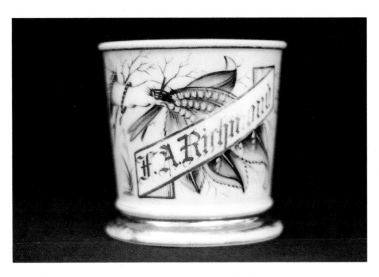

Hand holding fern. *Courtesy of Dr. Ralph Nix.*

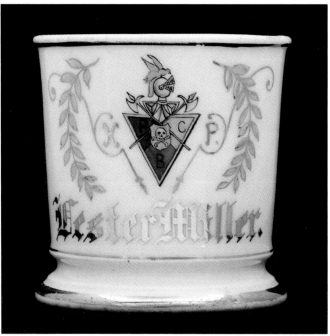

Knights of Pythias, (K. of P.). *Anonymous.*

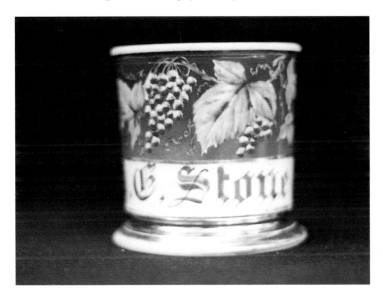

Currants. *Courtesy of Dr. Ralph Nix.*

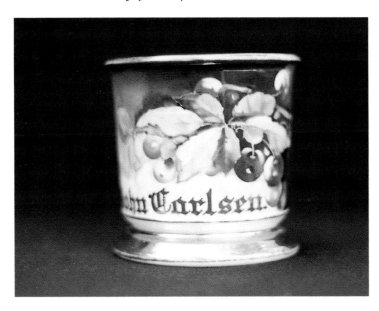

Cherries. *Courtesy of Dr. Ralph Nix.*

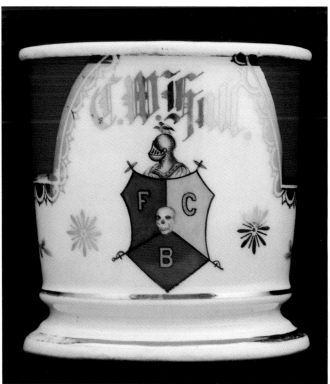

K. of P. *Courtesy of Anthony Gugliotti.*

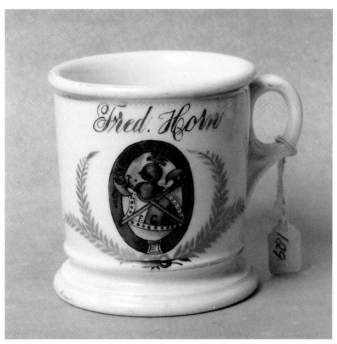

K. of P., preferred example. *Courtesy of David Giese.*

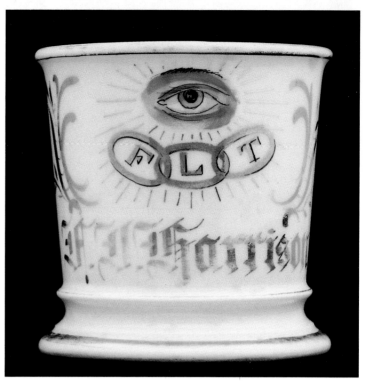

Odd Fellows. *Courtesy of Anthony Gugliotti.*

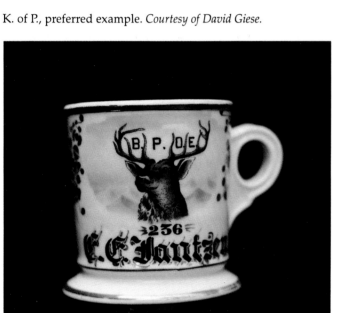

B.P.O.E. (Elks). *Courtesy of Bernard Lukco.*

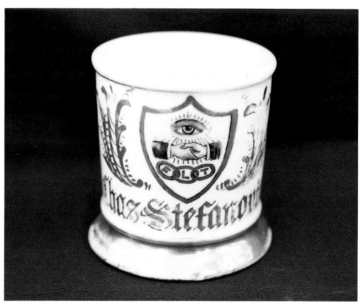

Odd Fellows. *Courtesy of Bernard Lukco.*

Odd Fellows, lodge designation, preferred example. *Courtesy of Bernard Lukco.*

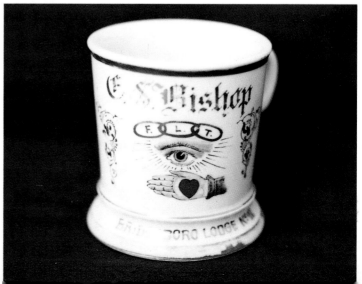

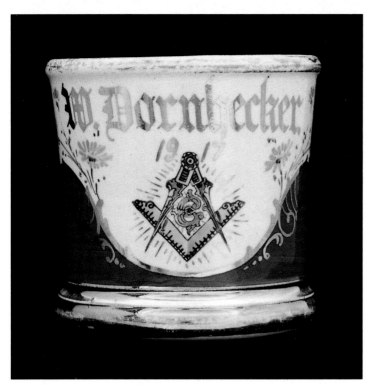

Mason. *Anonymous.*

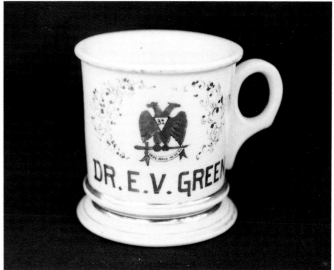

Mason, 32nd degree arch mason. *Courtesy of Bernard Lukco.*

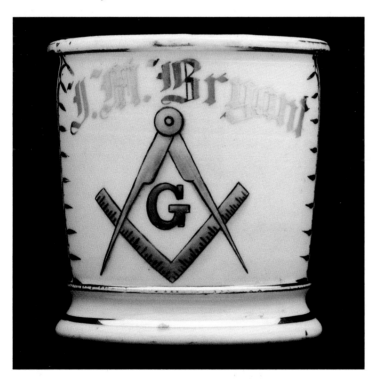

Mason. *Courtesy of Anthony Gugliotti.*

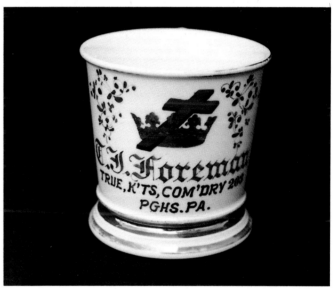

Knight Templar, lodge designation. *Courtesy of Bernard Lukco.*

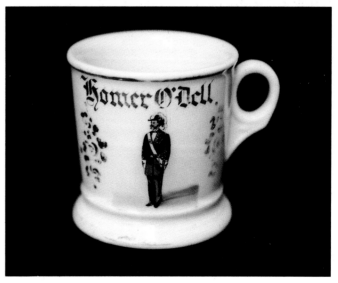

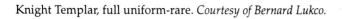

Knight Templar, full uniform-rare. *Courtesy of Bernard Lukco.*

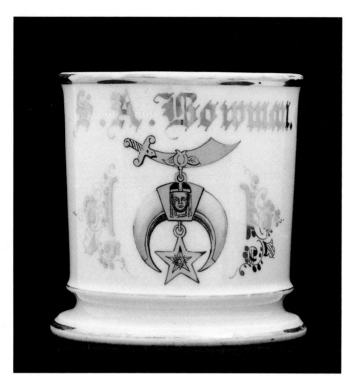

Mystic shrine. *Anonymous.*

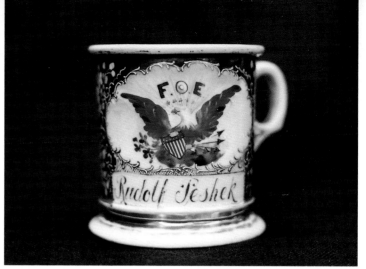

F.O.E., preferred example. *Courtesy of Bernard Lukco.*

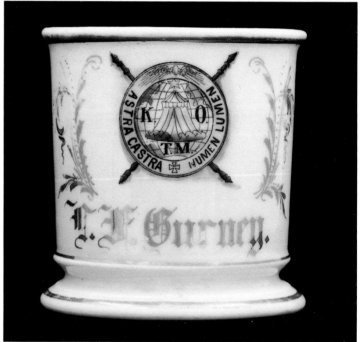

Knights of Tented Maccabees. *Anonymous.*

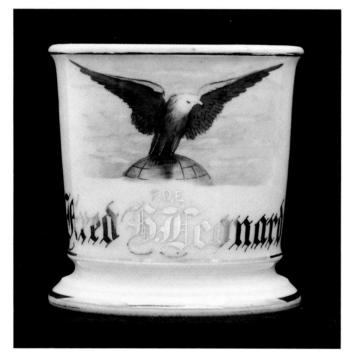

Fraternal Order of Eagles (FOE). *Anonymous.*

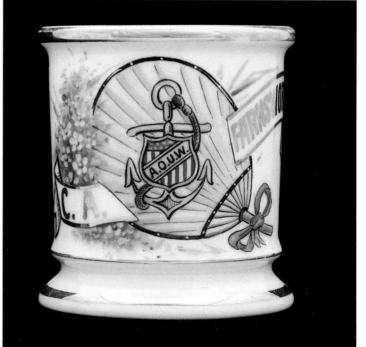

Ancient Order of United Workmen, (AOUW). "Fancy" example. *Anonymous.*

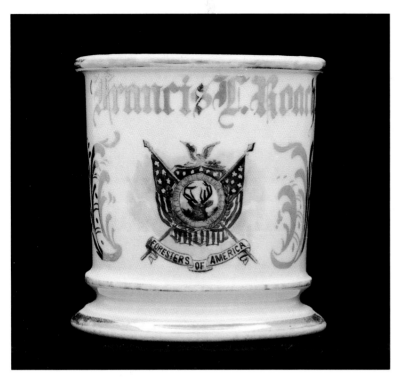

Foresters of America. *Anonymous.*

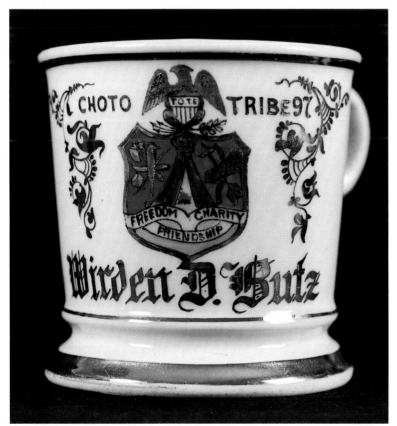

Order of Redmen, tribe number. *Courtesy of Morris Pickerell, Jr.*

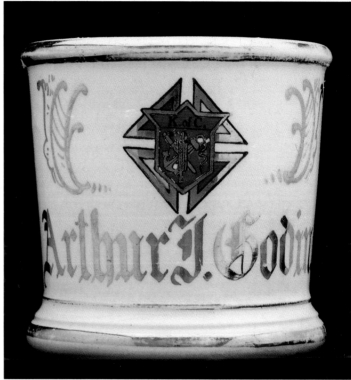

Knights of Columbus. *Courtesy of Anthony Gugliotti.*

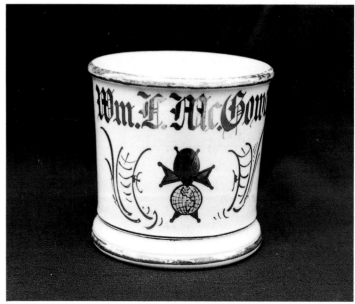

Knights of Columbus, 4th degree. *Courtesy of Bernard Lukco.*

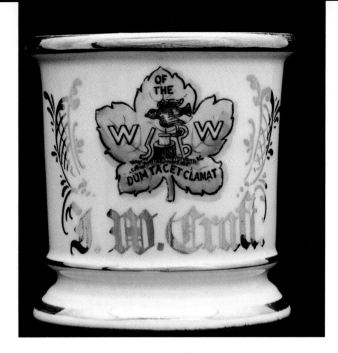

Woodmen of the World, green leaf. *Anonymous.*

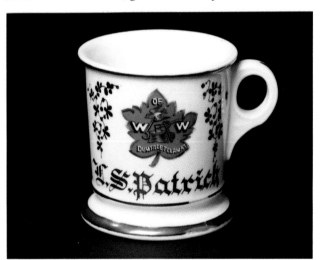

Woodmen of the World, blue leaf. *Courtesy of Thomas and Penelope Nader.*

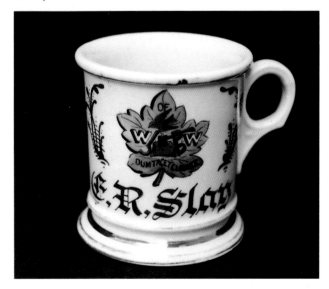

W.O.W., multi-color leaf. *Courtesy of Bernard Lukco.*

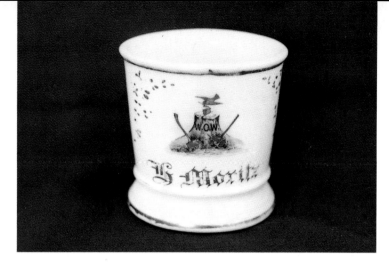

W.O.W., stump, ax and bird. *Courtesy of Bernard Lukco.*

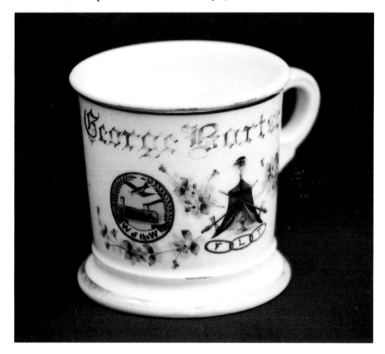

W.O.W. and Odd Fellow Double Fraternal. *Courtesy of Bernard Lukco.*

Patriotic Order of the Sons of America (P.O.S. of A.). *Anonymous.*

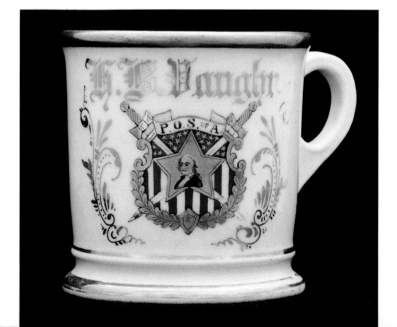

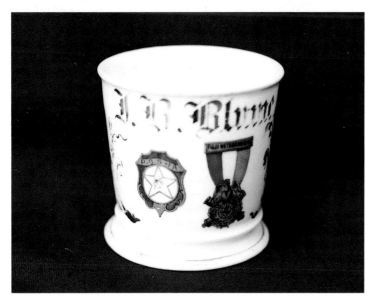

P.O.S. of A., Sons of Veterans-Double Fraternal. *Courtesy of Bernard Lukco.*

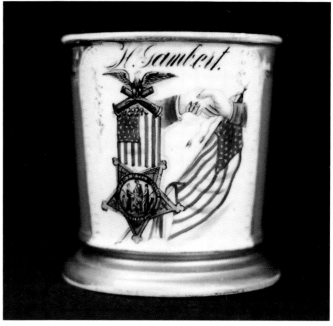

G.A.R., Union and Confederate handshake, rare. *Courtesy of Dr. Ralph Nix.*

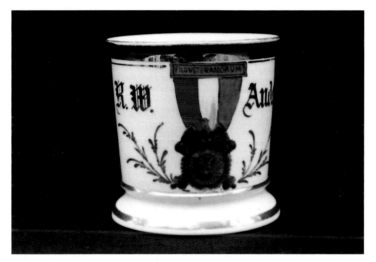

Sons of Veterans. *Courtesy of Bernard Lukco.*

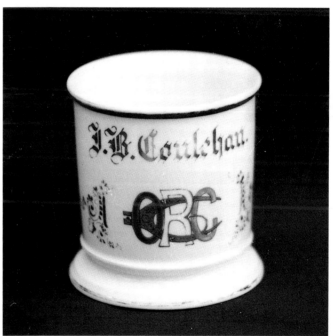

Order of Rail Road Conductors (ticket punch). *Courtesy of Bernard Lukco.*

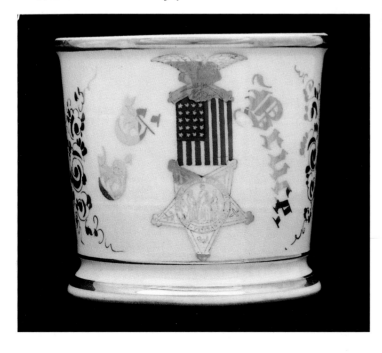

Grand Army of the Republic (G.A.R.). *Anonymous.*

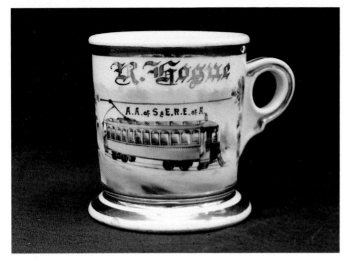

Amalgamated Association of Streetcar and Electric Railway Employees of America. *Courtesy of Bernard Lukco.*

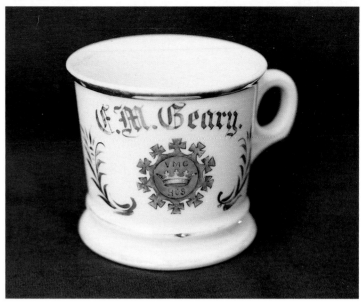

Royal Arcanum. *Courtesy of Bernard Lukco.*

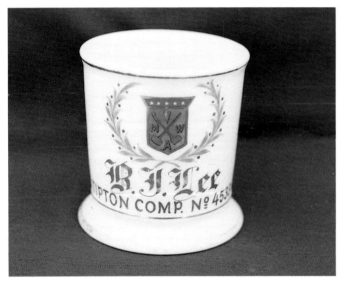

Modern Woodmen of America (MWA). *Courtesy of Bernard Lukco.*

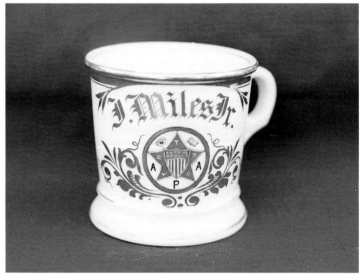

American Protective Association. *Courtesy of Bernard Lukco.*

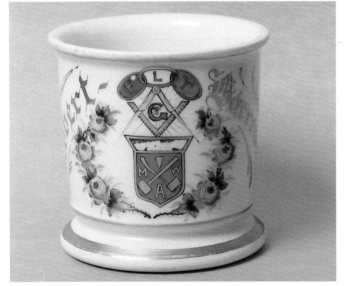

Triple Emblem, M.W.A., Mason and Odd Fellow. *Courtesy of David Giese.*

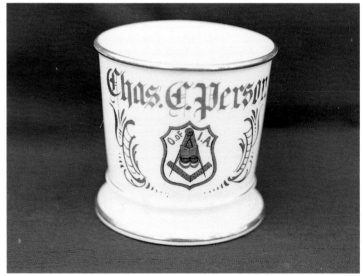

Order of Independent Americans. *Courtesy of Bernard Lukco.*

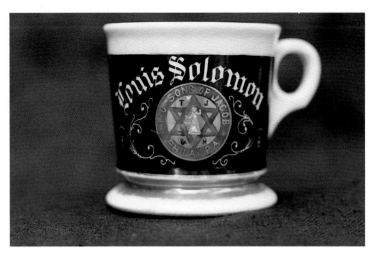

Sons of Jacob. *Courtesy of Bernard Lukco.*

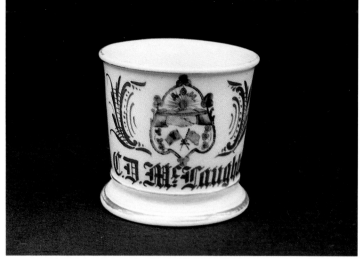

A.O.H., large design. *Courtesy of Bernard Lukco.*

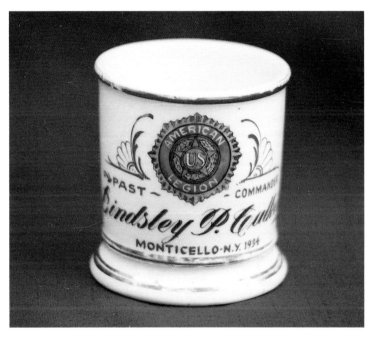

American Legion. *Courtesy of Bernard Lukco.*

Ancient Order of Hibernians (A.O.H.). *Anonymous.*

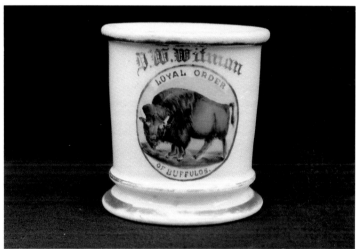

Loyal Order of Buffalos. *Courtesy of Bernard Lukco.*

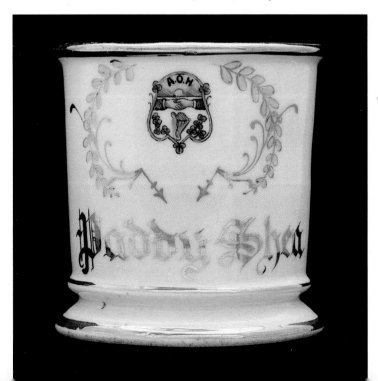

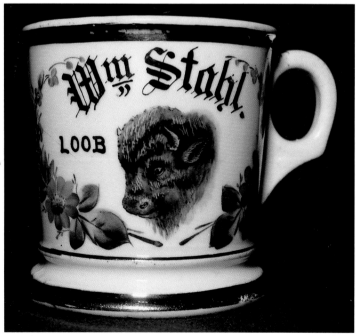

Loyal Order of Buffalos. *Courtesy of Raymond and Theresa Jones.*

69

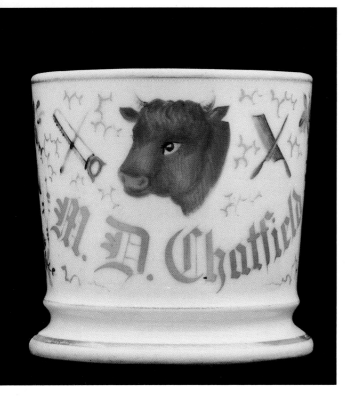

Steer head. *Courtesy of Anthony Gugliotti.*

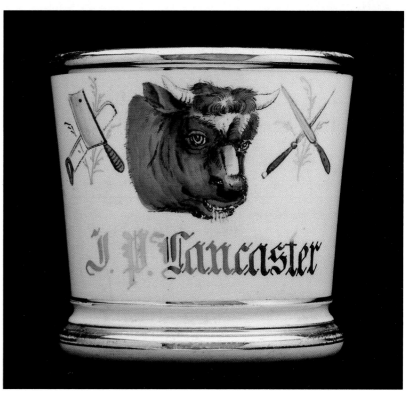

Steer head. *Courtesy of Anthony Gugliotti.*

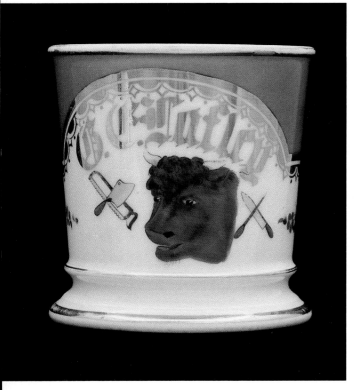

Steer head. *Anonymous.*

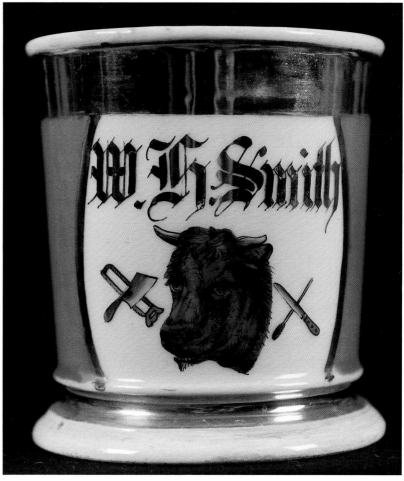

Steer head. *Courtesy of Morris Pickerell, Jr.*

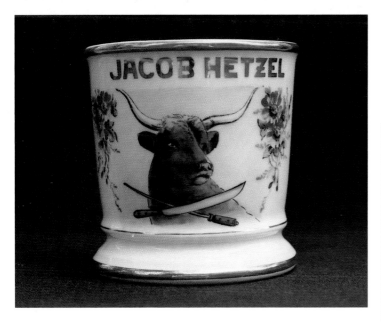

Steer head. *Courtesy of Dr. Ralph Nix.*

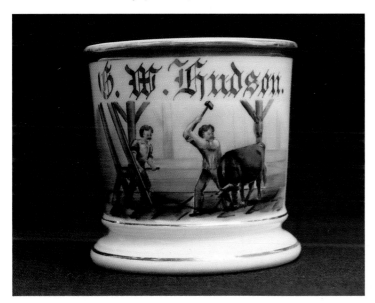

Slaughterhouse. *Courtesy of Dr. Ralph Nix.*

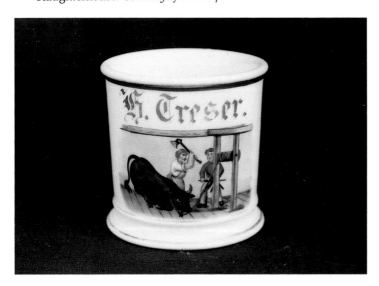

Slaughterhouse. *Courtesy of Bernard Lukco.*

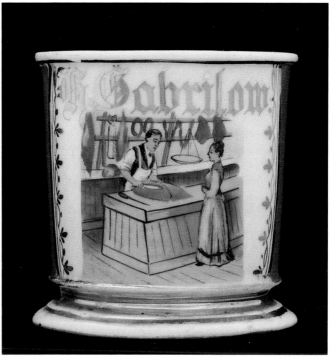

Meat market. *Anonymous.*

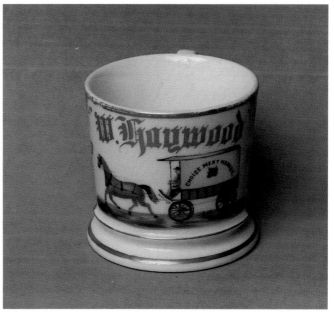

Meat market wagon. *Courtesy of David Giese.*

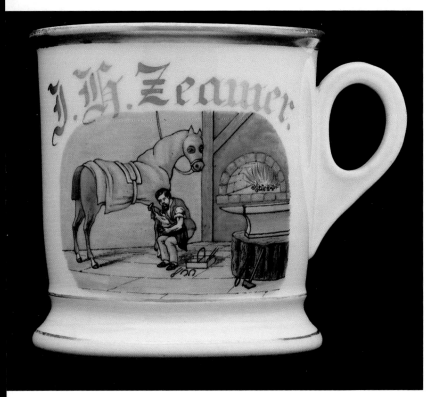

Blacksmith working. *Courtesy of Anthony Gugliotti.*

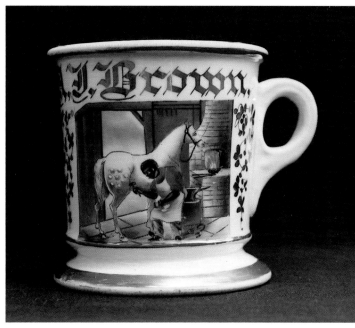

Afro-American blacksmith, rare. *Courtesy of Dr. Ralph Nix.*

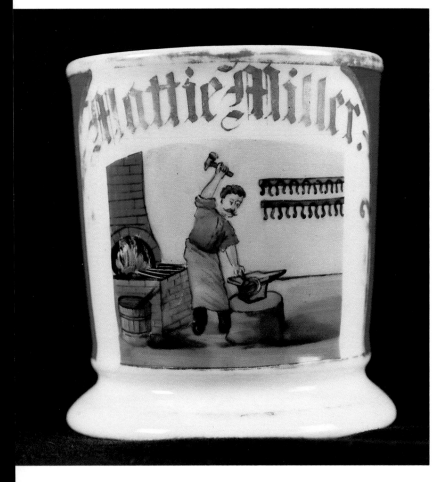

Blacksmith with anvil. *Courtesy of Morris Pickerell, Jr.*

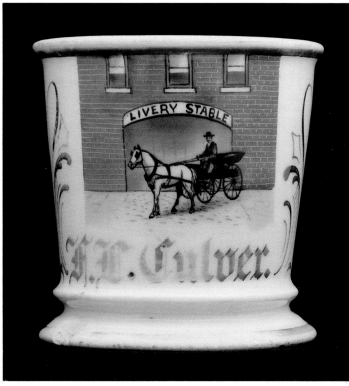

Livery stable. *Courtesy of Anthony Gugliotti.*

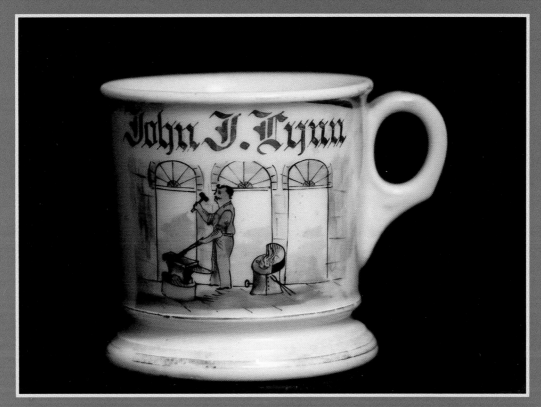

Wrought iron blacksmith. *Courtesy of Michael J. Griffin.*

Bartender

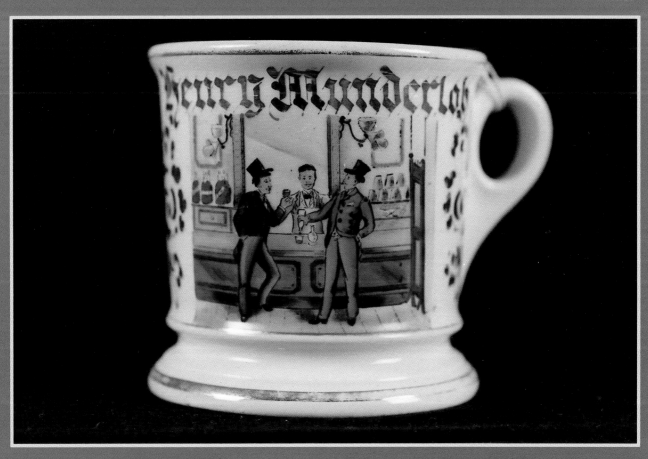

Bartender. *Courtesy of Morris Pickerell, Jr.*

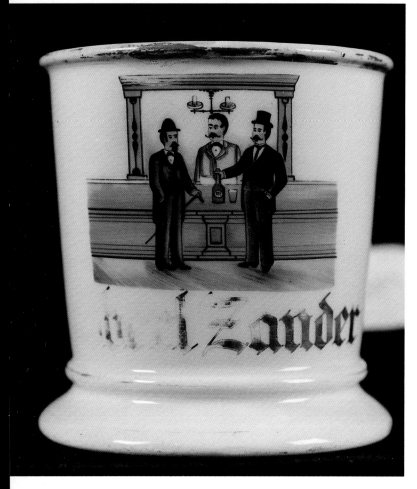

Bartender, *Courtesy of Morris Pickerell, Jr.*

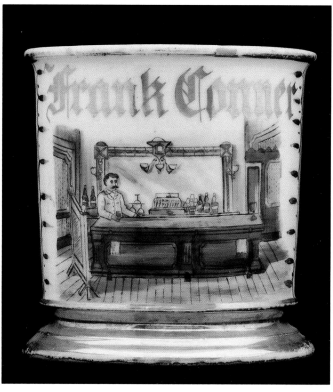

Bartender, alone. *Courtesy of Anthony Gugliotti.*

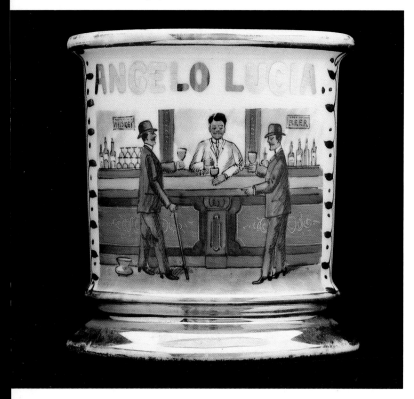

Bartender, details.*Courtesy of Anthony Gugliotti.*

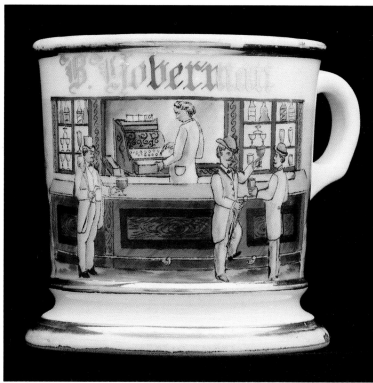

Bartender, details. *Courtesy of Anthony Gugliotti.*

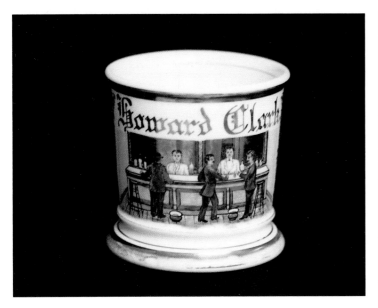

Two Bartenders. *Courtesy of Roland F. Porter.*

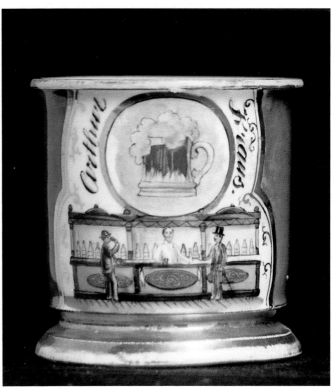

Bartender, glass of beer above, rare. *Courtesy of Michael J. Griffin.*

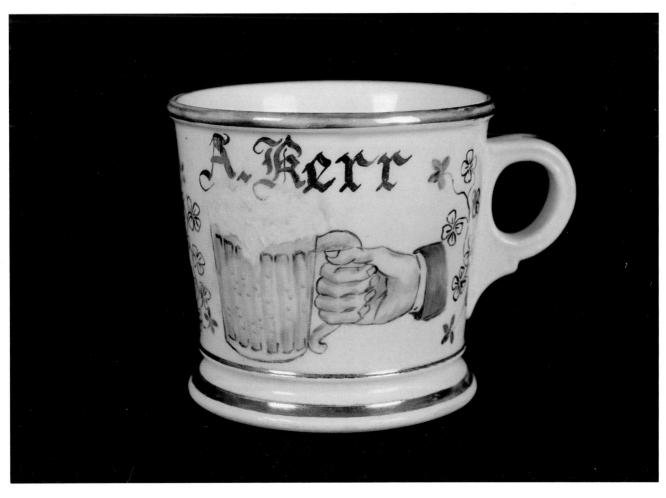

Glass of beer. *Courtesy of Morris Pickerell, Jr.*

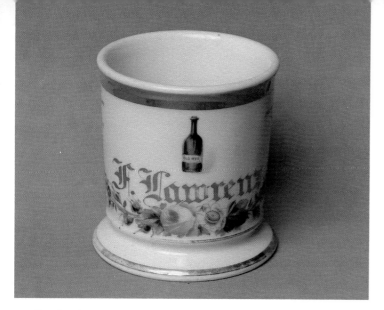

Bottle of rye. *Courtesy of David Giese.*

Brewers

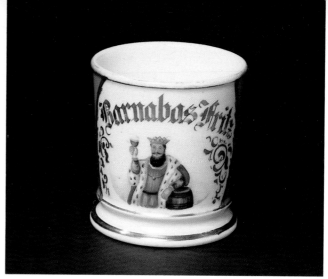

Brewmaster (Gambrinus). *Courtesy of Thomas and Penelope Nader.*

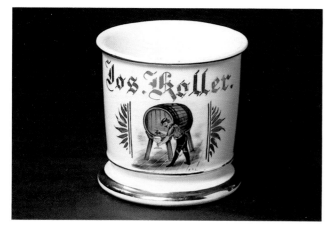

Beer cellar. *Courtesy of Thomas and Penelope Nader.*

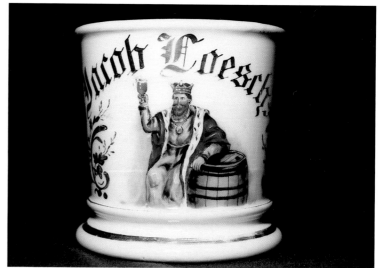

Brewmaster (Gambrinus). *Courtesy of Raymond and Theresa Jones.*

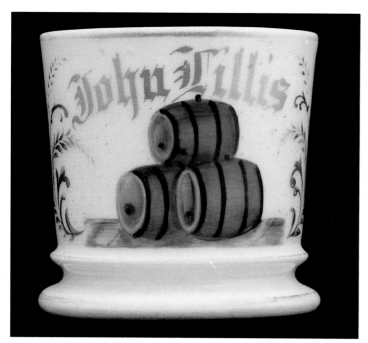

Beer barrels. *Courtesy of Anthony Gugliotti.*

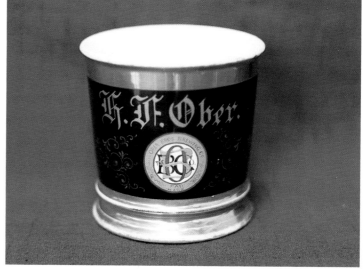

Brewery Owner, Ober Brothers Brewing company. *Courtesy of Bernard Lukco.*

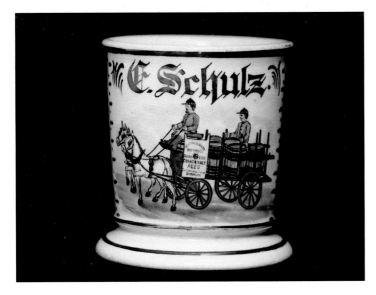

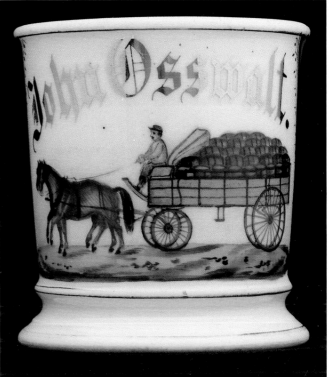

Brewery wagon, New York and Brooklyn Brewing Company. *Courtesy of Michael J. Griffin.*

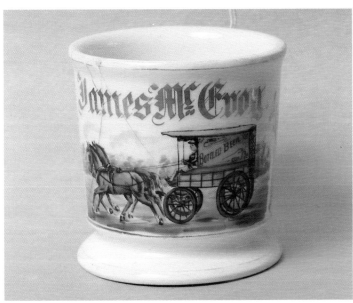

Brewery wagon, driver's cover down. *Courtesy of Anthony Gugliotti.*

Cowboys and Cattlemen

Bottled beer wagon. *Courtesy of David Giese.*

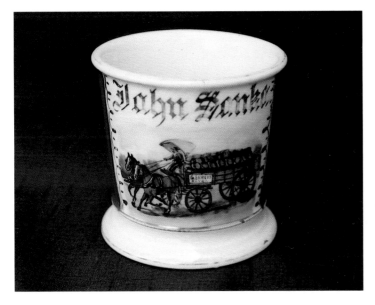

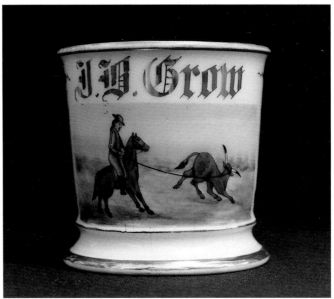

Brewery wagon, driver's cover up. *Courtesy of Bernard Lukco.*

Cowboy roping steer. *Courtesy of Dr. Ralph Nix.*

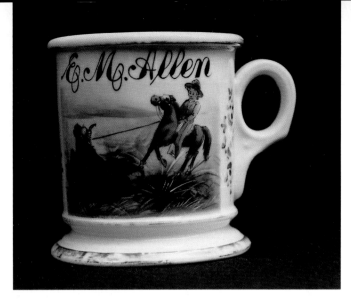

Cowboy roping steer. *Courtesy of Dr. Ralph Nix.*

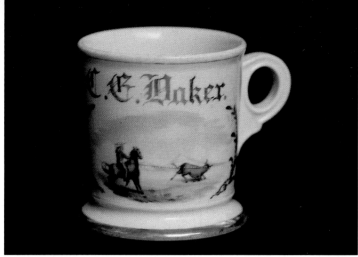

Cowboy, long hair, roping steer. *Courtesy of Roland F. Porter.*

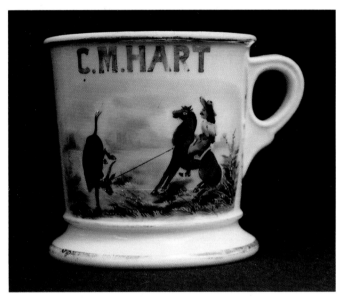

Cowboy roping steer. *Courtesy of Dr. Ralph Nix.*

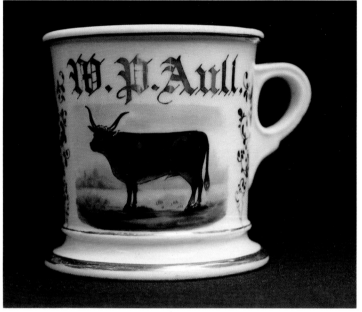

Cattleman, long horn steer. *Courtesy of Dr. Ralph Nix.*

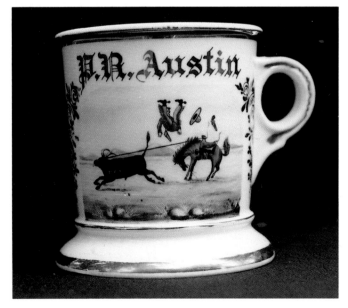

Cowboy bucked from horse, rare. *Courtesy of Dr. Ralph Nix.*

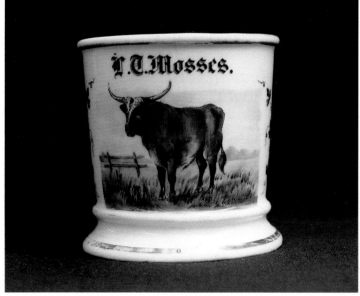

Cattleman, long horn steer. *Courtesy of Dr. Ralph Nix.*

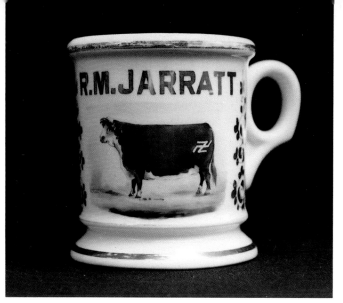

Cattleman, steer with brand. *Courtesy of Dr. Ralph Nix.*

The Dairy

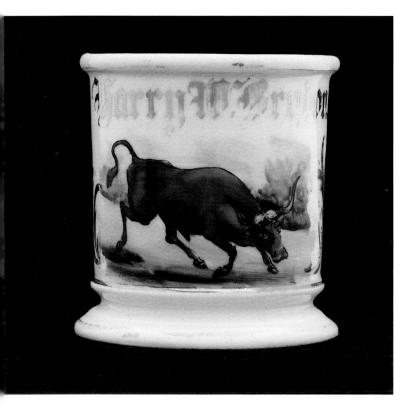

Cattleman, long horn steer charging. *Anonymous.*

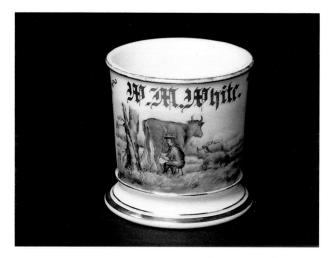

Dairy farmer. *Courtesy of Thomas and Penelope Nader.*

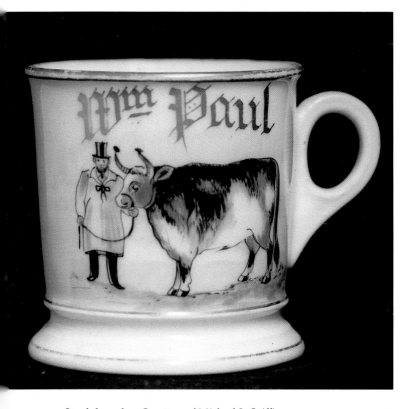

Stock breeder. *Courtesy of Michael J. Griffin.*

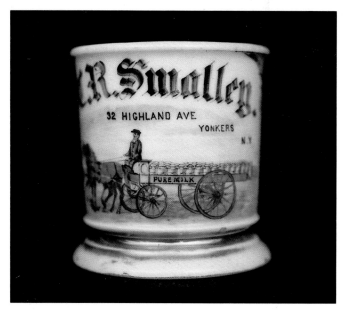

Farm milk wagon, Yonkers, New York. *Courtesy of Charles F. Kalb.*

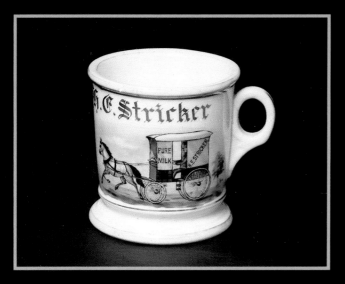

Milk wagon. *Courtesy of Thomas and Penelope Nader.*

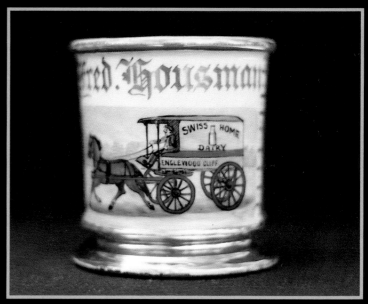

Dairy wagon, swiss home dairy. *Courtesy of Dr. Ralph Nix.*

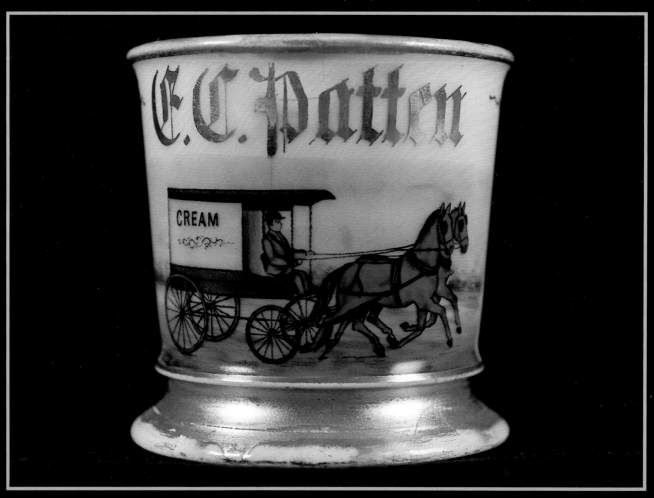

Cream wagon. *Courtesy of Morris Pickerell, Jr.*

The Dentist

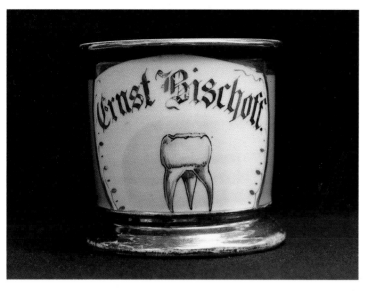

Molar. *Courtesy of Dr. Ralph Nix.*

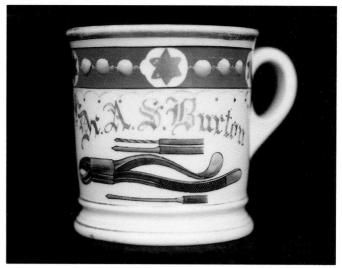

Dentist tools. *Courtesy of Charles F. Kalb.*

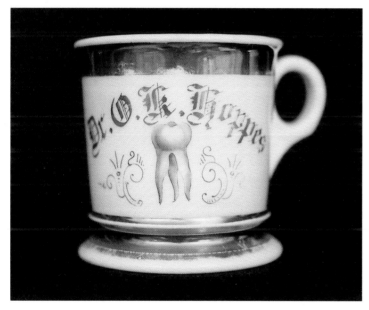

Molar, doctor. *Courtesy of Charles F. Kalb.*

Dentist, occupational by courtesy. *Courtesy of Dr. Ralph Nix.*

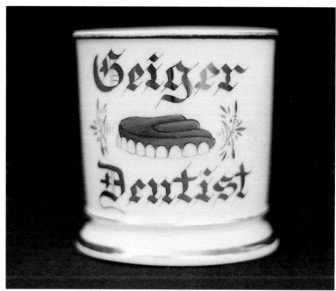

False teeth. *Courtesy of Dr. Ralph Nix.*

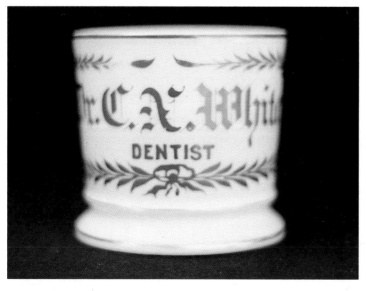

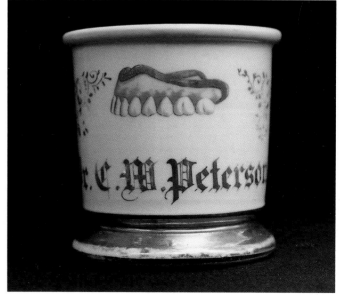

False teeth, doctor. *Courtesy of Dr. Ralph Nix.*

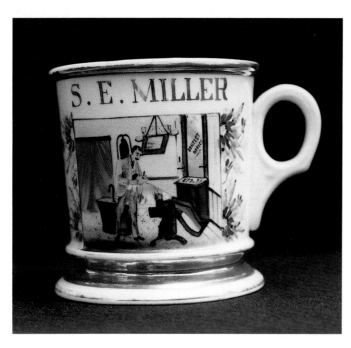

Working dentist. *Courtesy of Dr. Ralph Nix.*

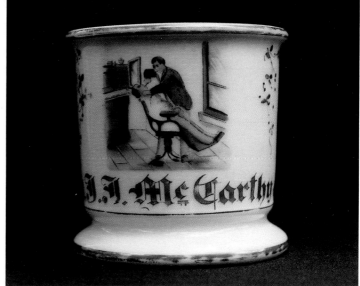

Working dentist. *Courtesy of Dr. Ralph Nix.*

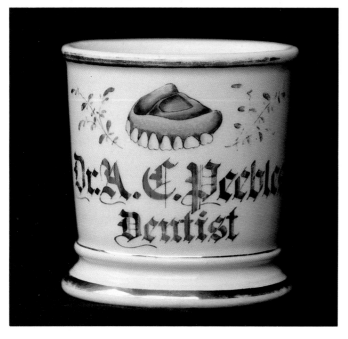

False teeth, doctor and dentist. *Anonymous.*

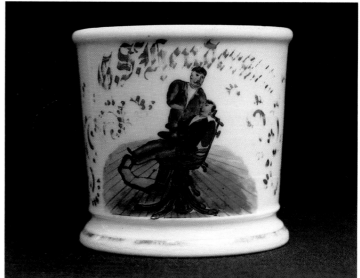

Working dentist. *Courtesy of Dr. Ralph Nix.*

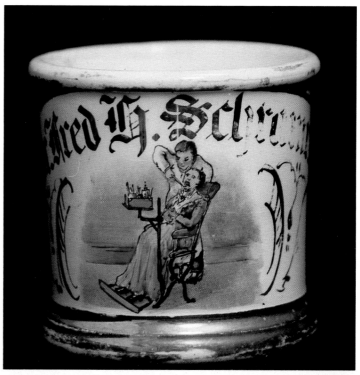

Working dentist, lady patient. *Courtesy of Michael J. Griffin.*

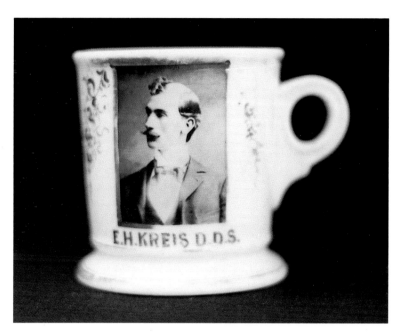

Photographic dentist. *Courtesy of Dr. Ralph Nix.*

Farm and Florist

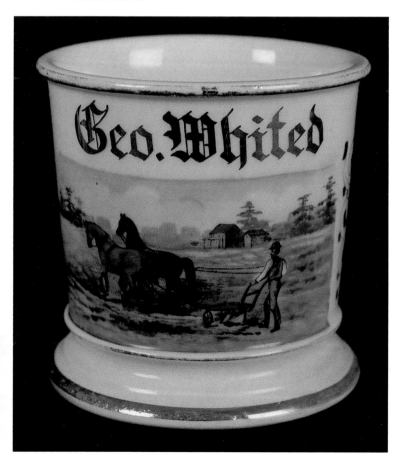

Farmer with plow. *Courtesy of Morris Pickerell, Jr.*

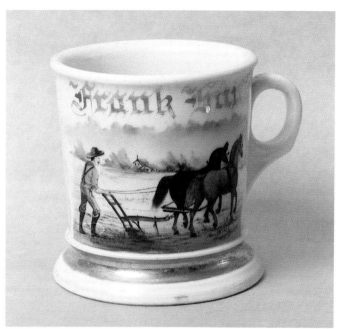

Farmer with plow. *Courtesy of David Giese.*

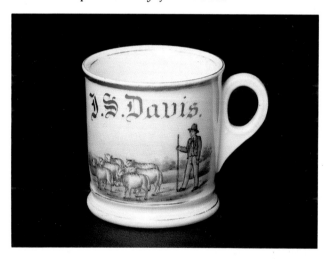

Shepherd. *Courtesy of Thomas and Penelope Nader.*

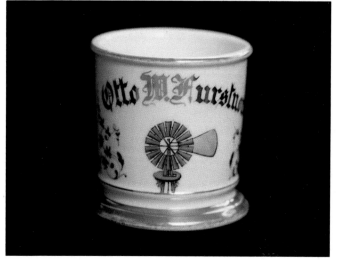

Farmer windmill. *Courtesy of Roland F. Porter.*

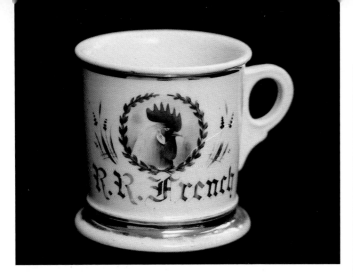

Rooster, poultry farmer. *Courtesy of Roland F. Porter.*

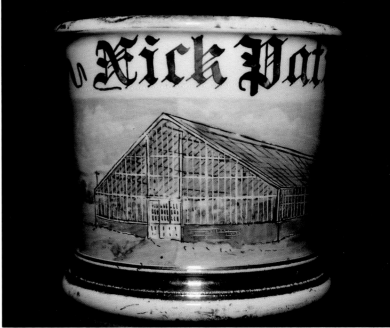

Greenhouse. *Courtesy of Raymond and Theresa Jones.*

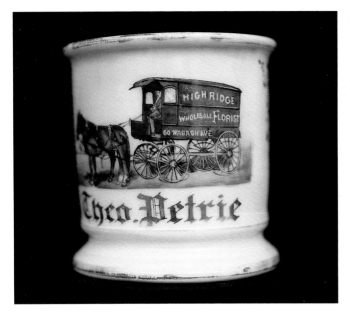

Wholesale florist wagon. *Courtesy of Charles F. Kalb.*

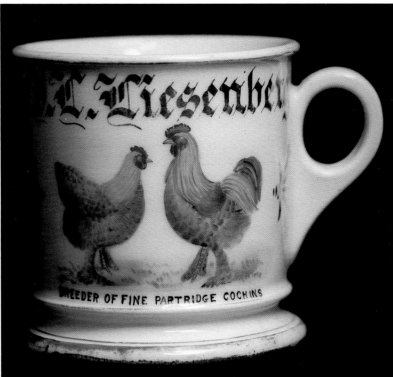

Poultry breeder, Cochins. *Courtesy of Michael J. Griffin.*

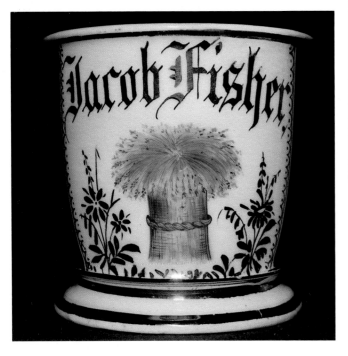

Wheat, farmer or grain dealer. *Courtesy of Raymond and Theresa Jones.*

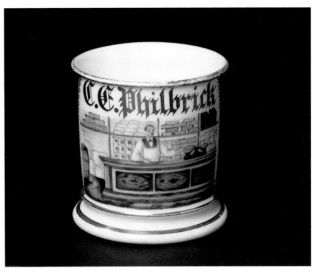

Grocery store, grocer only. *Courtesy of Thomas and Penelope Nader.*

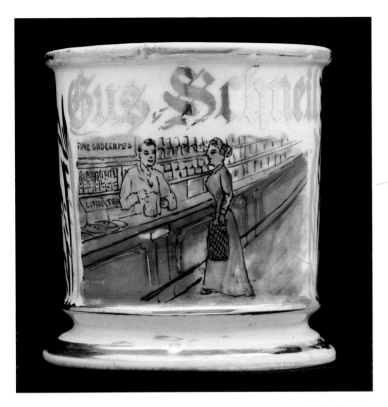

Grocery store. *Courtesy of Anthony Gugliotti.*

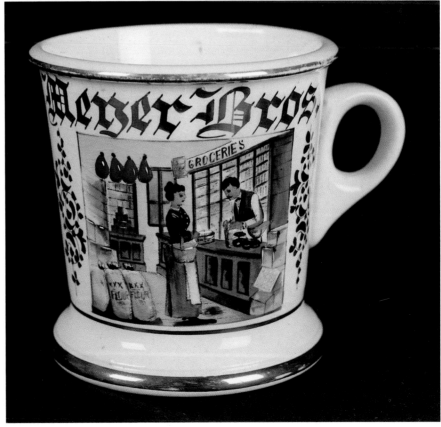

Grocery store. *Courtesy of Morris Pickerell, Jr.*

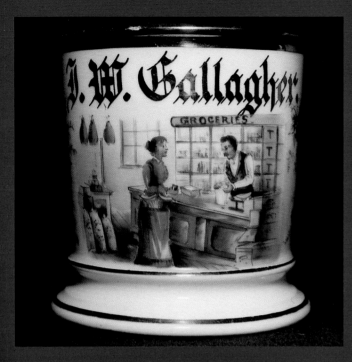

Grocery store. *Courtesy of Raymond and Theresa Jones.*

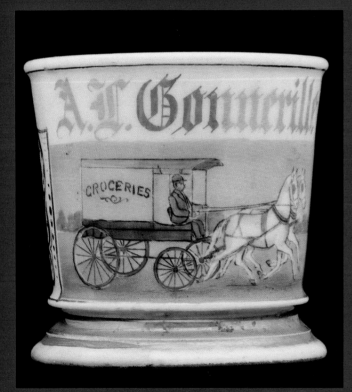

Grocery wagon. *Courtesy of Anthony Gugliotti.*

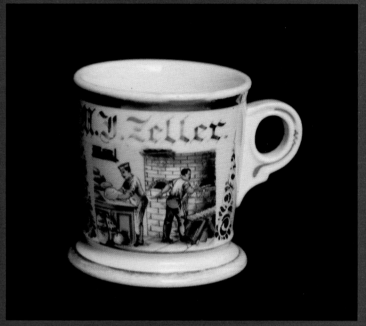

Bakers. *Courtesy of Roland F. Porter.*

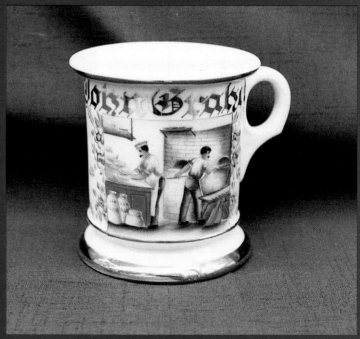

Bakers. *Courtesy of Bernard Lukco.*

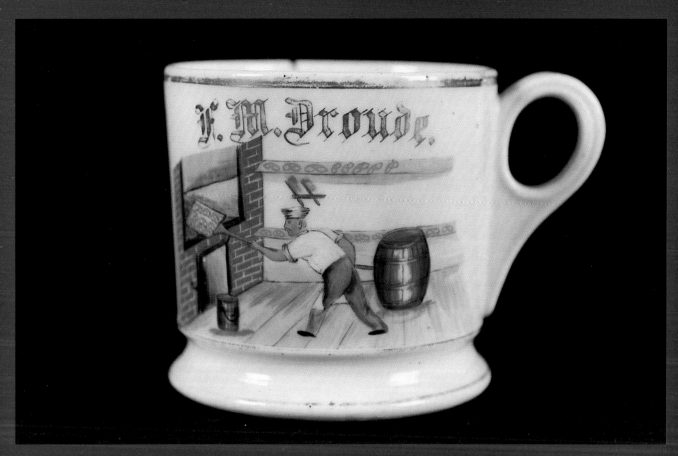

Pretzel baker. *Courtesy of Morris Pickerell, Jr.*

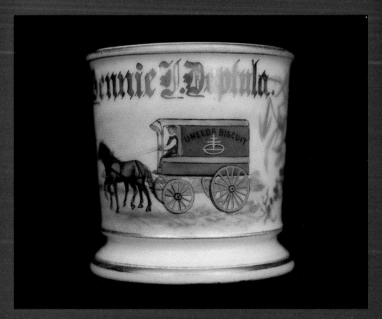

Biscuit wagon. *Courtesy of Charles F. Kalb.*

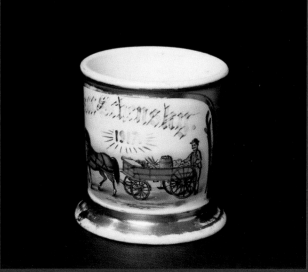

Vegetable huckster. *Courtesy of Thomas and Penelope Nader.*

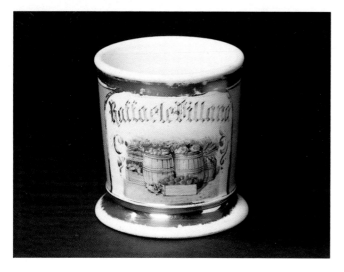

Produce dealer. *Courtesy of Thomas and Penelope Nader.*

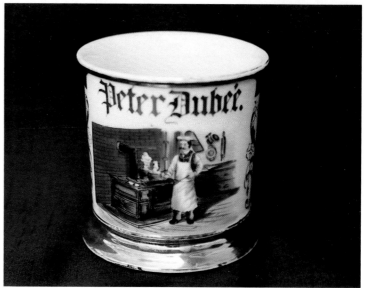

Chef or cook. *Courtesy of Bernard Lukco.*

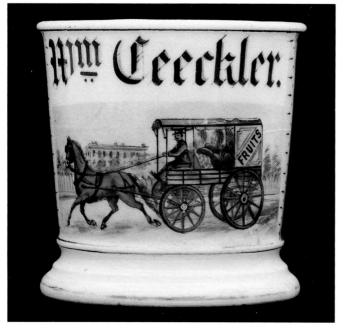

Fruit wagon. *Anonymous.*

Food Service

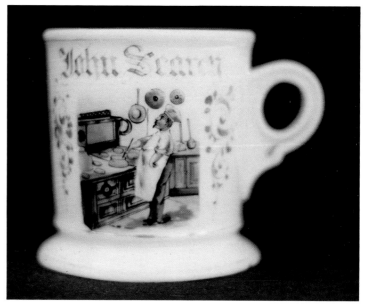

Chef. *Courtesy of Dr. Ralph Nix.*

Chef, holding platter. *Anonymous.*

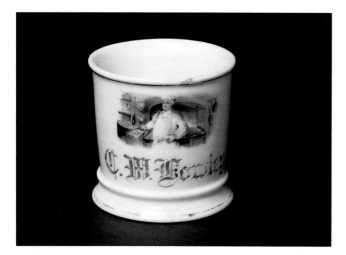

Chef. *Courtesy of Thomas and Penelope Nader.*

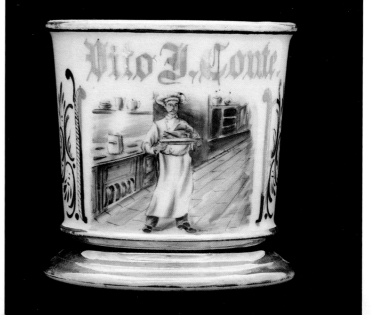

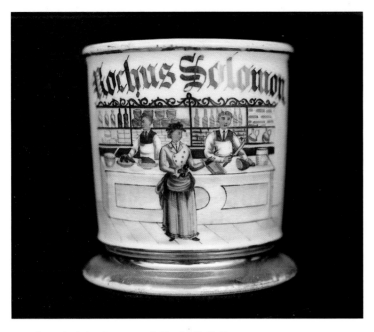

Jewish deli. *Courtesy of Charles F. Kalb.*

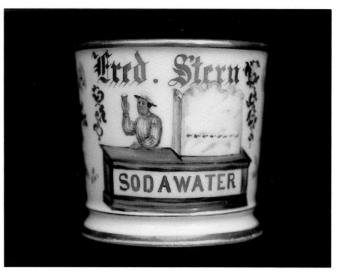

Soda fountain. *Courtesy of Charles F. Kalb.*

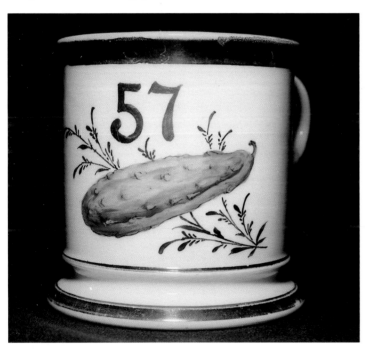

Pickle dealer. *Courtesy of Raymond and Theresa Jones.*

Confectioner. *Courtesy of Thomas and Penelope Nader.*

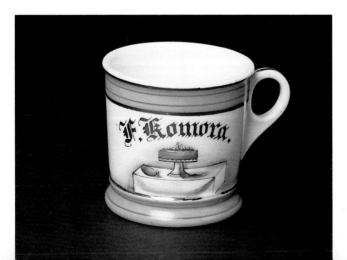

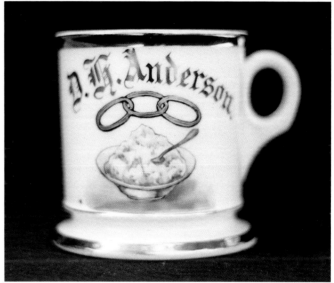

Occu-Frat, ice cream parlor, with Odd Fellow symbol. *Courtesy of Dr. Ralph Nix.*

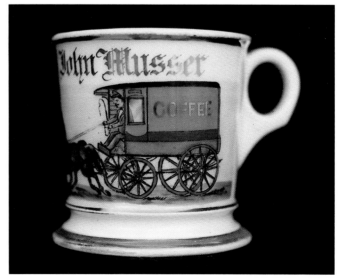

Coffee wagon. *Courtesy of Charles F. Kalb.*

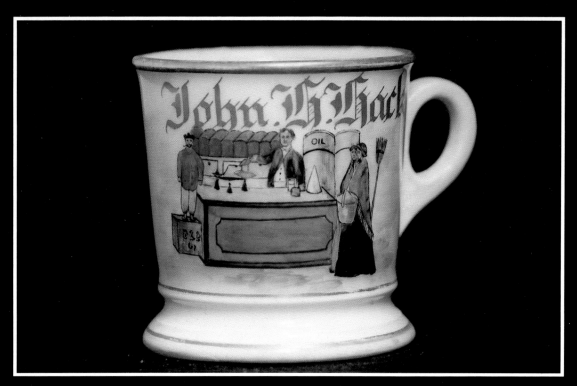

Tea store, wooden Chinese man advertising. *Courtesy of Michael J. Griffin.*

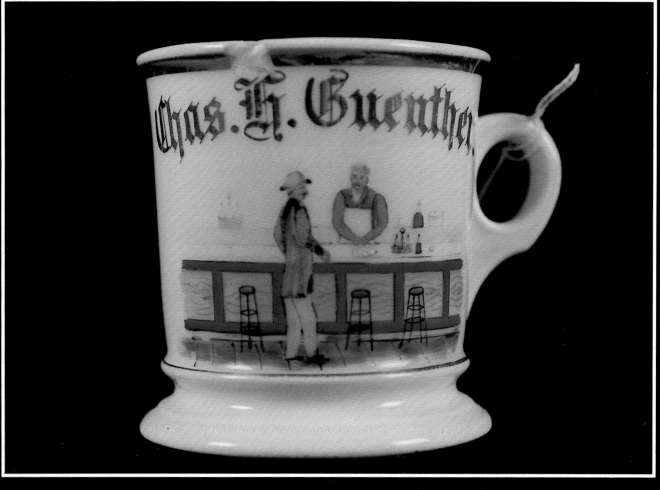

Oyster bar. *Courtesy of Morris Pickerell, Jr.*

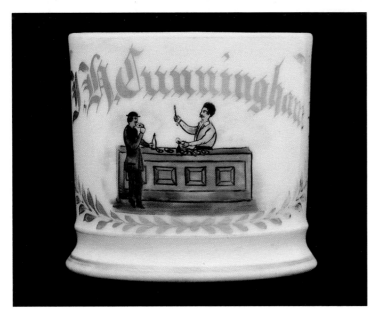

Oyster bar. *Anonymous.*

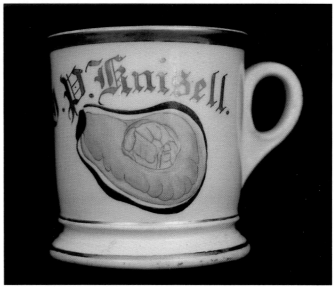

Oyster. *Courtesy of Charles F. Kalb.*

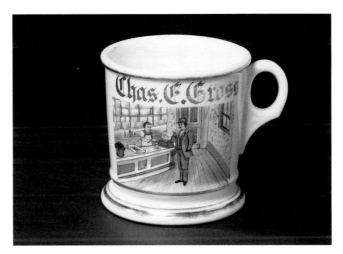

Oyster bar, ice on oysters. *Courtesy of Thomas and Penelope Nader.*

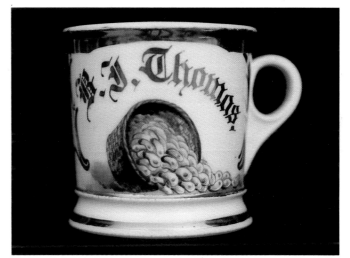

Basket of oysters. *Courtesy of Charles F. Kalb.*

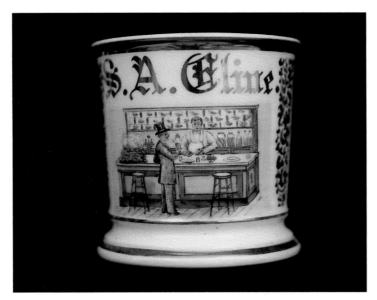

Oyster bar, ice on oysters. *Courtesy of Charles F. Kalb.*

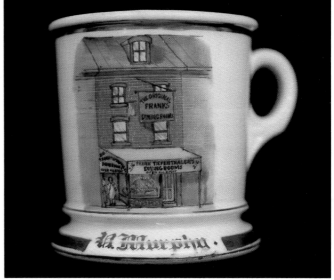

Seafood restaurant, Frank's of Philadelphia. *Courtesy of Charles F. Kalb.*

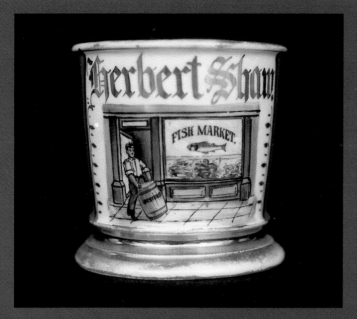

Fish market. *Courtesy of Charles F. Kalb.*

Footwear, hats and garments

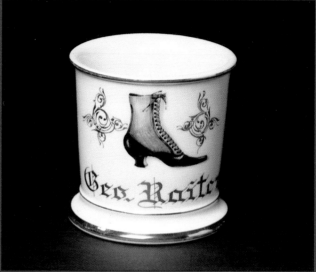

Ladies' shoemaker. *Courtesy of Thomas and Penelope Nader.*

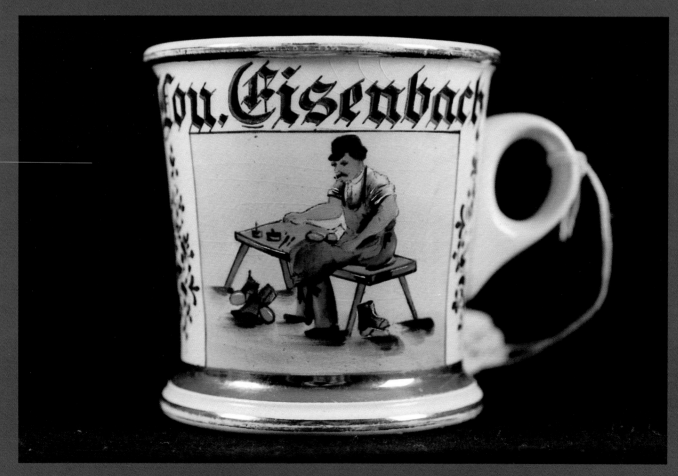

Cobbler. *Courtesy of Morris Pickerell, Jr.*

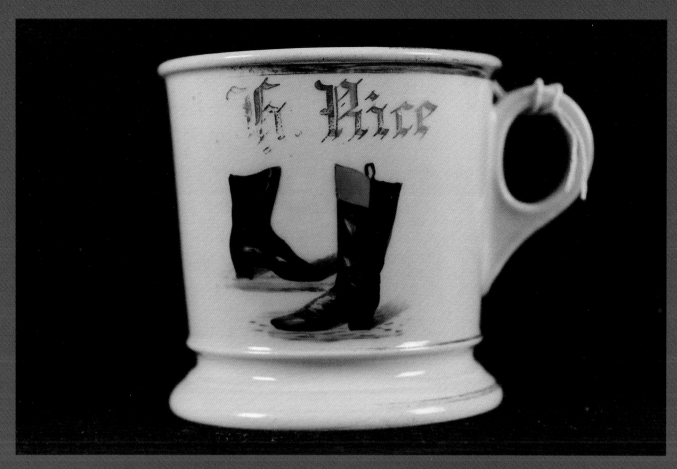

Bootmaker. *Courtesy of Morris Pickerell, Jr.*

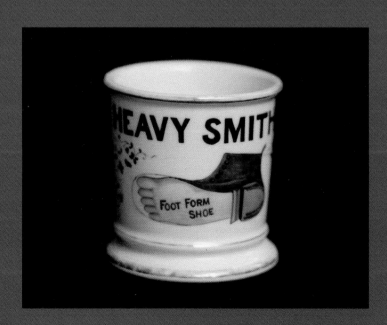

Footform shoe, heavy smith. *Courtesy of Roland F. Porter.*

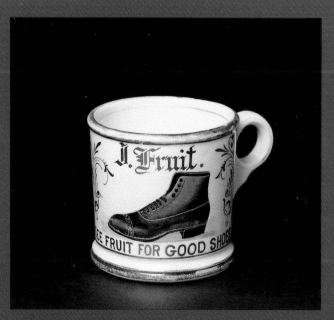

Shoe salesman. *Courtesy of Thomas and Penelope Nader.*

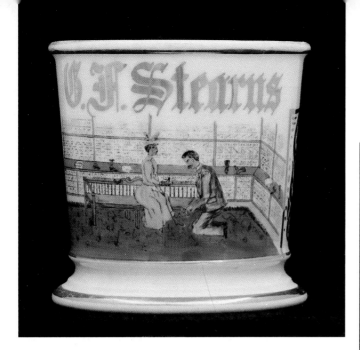

Shoe store. *Anonymous.*

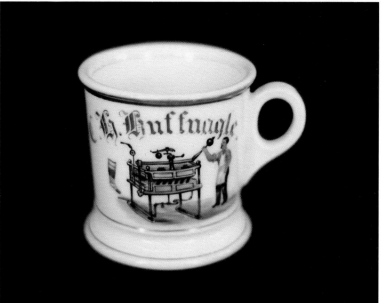

Sock making machine. *Courtesy of Bernard Lukco.*

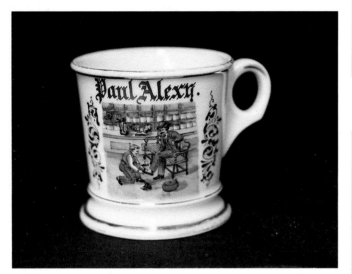

Shoe store, male customer. *Courtesy of Bernard Lukco.*

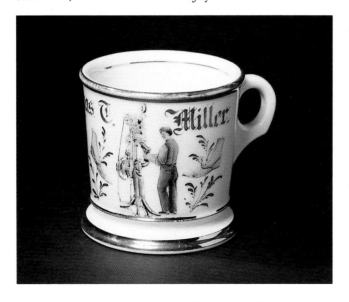

Shoe making machine. *Courtesy of Thomas and Penelope Nader.*

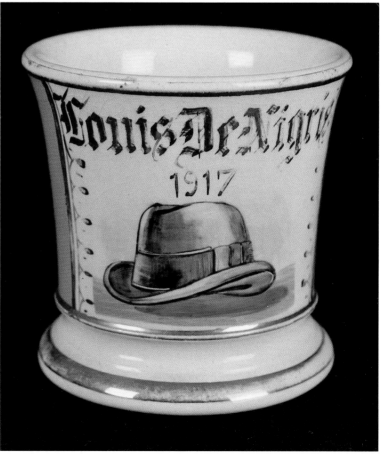

Hat maker. *Courtesy of Morris Pickerell, Jr.*

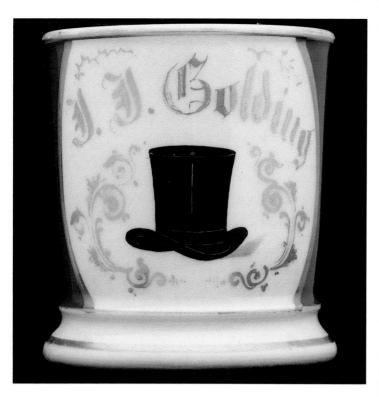

Top hat. *Courtesy of Anthony Gugliotti.*

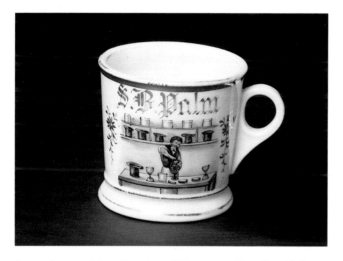

Hat maker, working. *Courtesy of Thomas and Penelope Nader.*

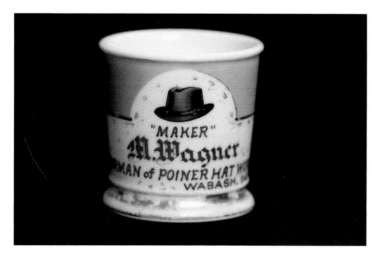

Foreman of Poiner Hat Factory. *Courtesy of Roland F. Porter.*

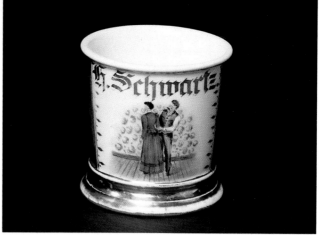

Dress maker. *Courtesy of Thomas and Penelope Nader.*

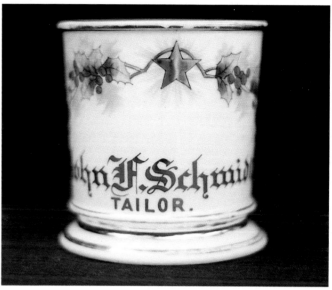

Tailor, occupation by courtesy. *Courtesy of Dr. Ralph Nix.*

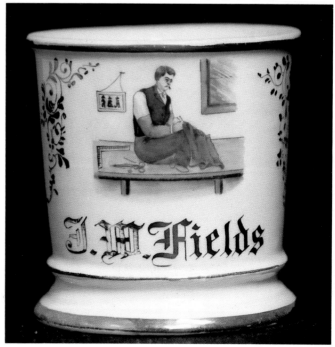

Tailor. *Courtesy of Michael J. Griffin.*

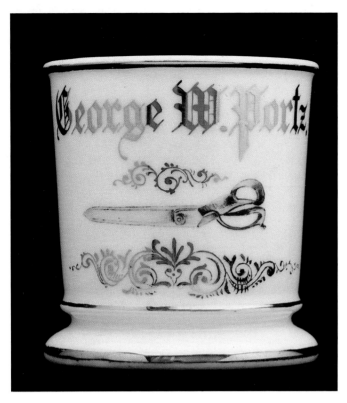

Fabric cutter. *Courtesy of Anthony Gugliotti.*

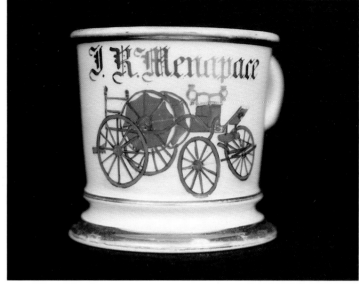

Hose cart. *Courtesy of Charles F. Kalb.*

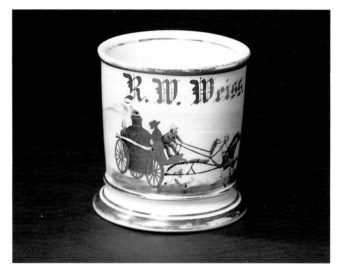

Steam pumper. *Courtesy of Thomas and Penelope Nader.*

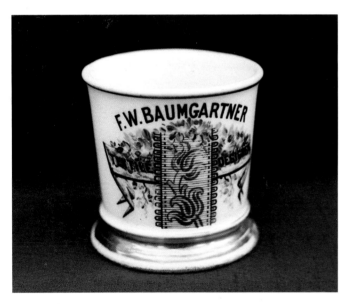

Textile designer. *Courtesy of Bernard Lukco.*

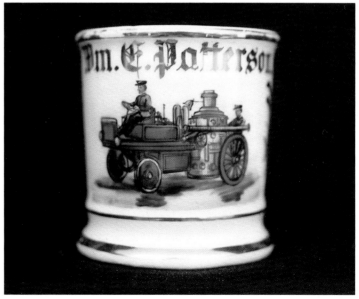

Motorized steam pumper. *Courtesy of Charles F. Kalb.*

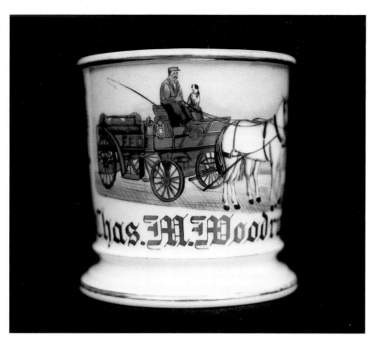

Utility wagon. *Courtesy of Charles F. Kalb.*

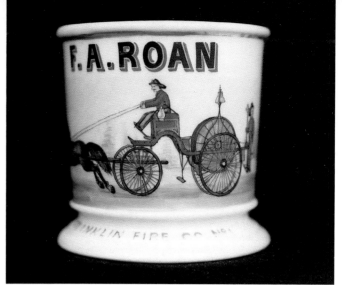

Hose cart. *Courtesy of Charles F. Kalb.*

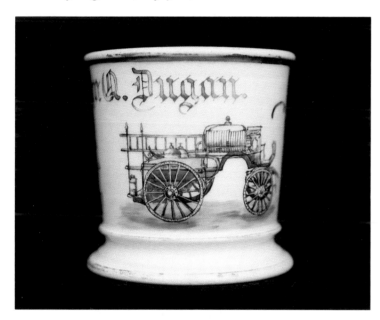

Chemical wagon. *Courtesy of Charles F. Kalb.*

Ladder wagon. *Courtesy of Charles F. Kalb.*

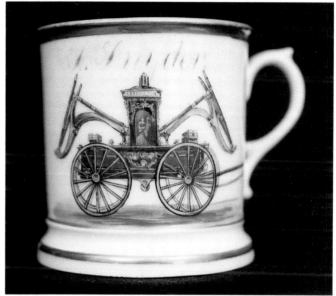

Kensington hand pumper. *Courtesy of Charles F. Kalb.*

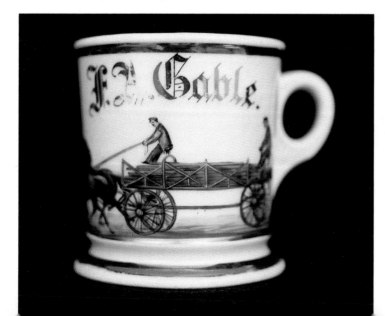

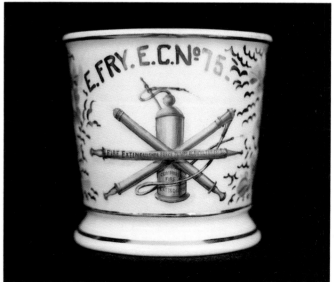

Fire extinguishers. *Courtesy of Charles F. Kalb.*

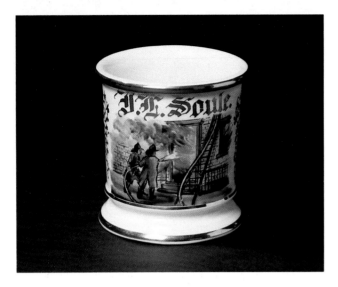

Firemen in action. *Courtesy of Thomas and Penelope Nader.*

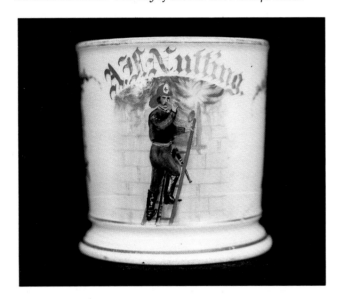

Fireman at window, Currier and Ives. *Courtesy of Charles F. Kalb.*

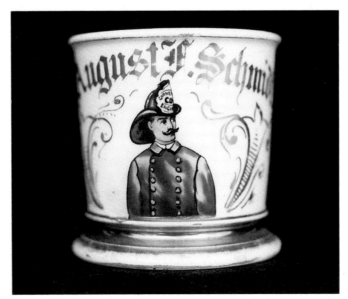

Fireman. *Courtesy of Charles F. Kalb.*

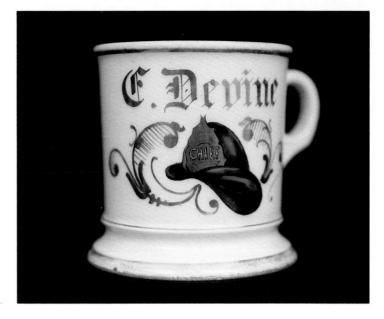

Fire chief's hat. *Courtesy of Charles F. Kalb.*

Law and Order

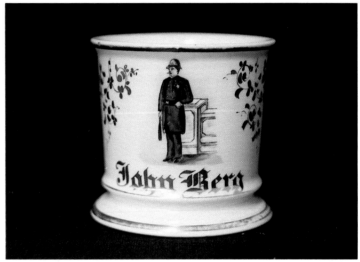

Policeman. *Courtesy of Bernard Lukco.*

Irish cop. *Courtesy of Charles F. Kalb.*

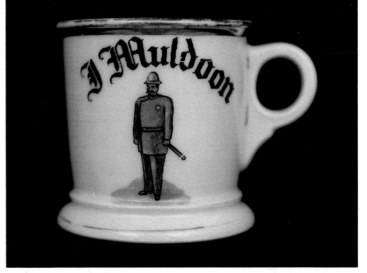

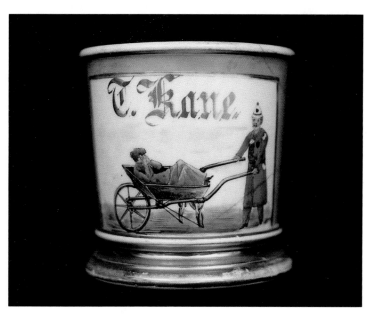

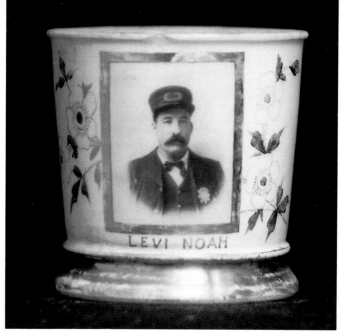

Cop taking a prostitute to jail in a wheel barrel, one of a kind. *Courtesy of Charles F. Kalb.*

Photographic deputy sheriff. *Courtesy of Michael J. Griffin.*

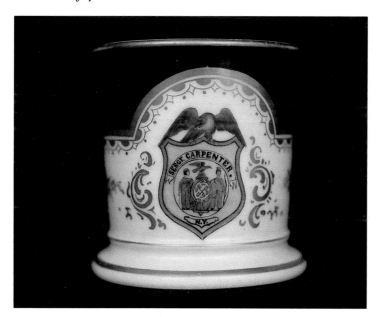

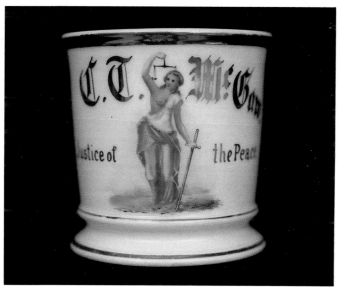

Justice of the Peace. *Courtesy of Charles F. Kalb.*

New York state police sergeant. *Courtesy of Charles F. Kalb.*

Judge in court room. *Courtesy of Charles F. Kalb.*

Federal marshall. *Courtesy of Charles F. Kalb.*

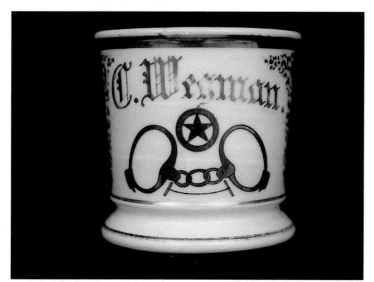

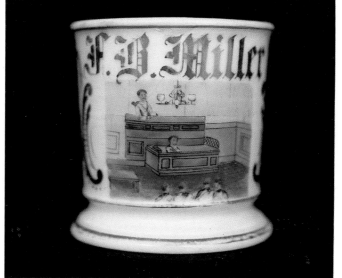

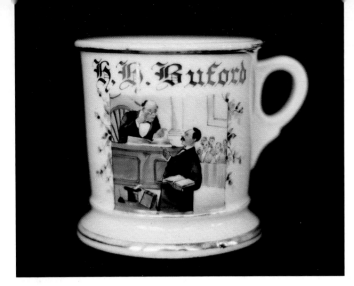

Lawyer. *Courtesy of Bernard Lukco.*

Life and Death

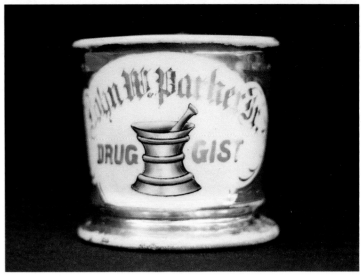

Doctor, mortar and pestle. *Courtesy of Dr. Ralph Nix.*

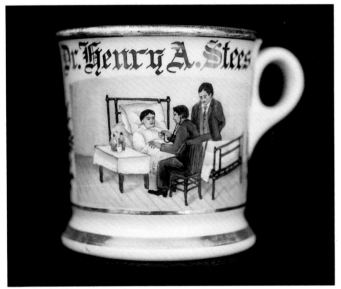

Doctor at bedside. *Courtesy of Charles F. Kalb.*

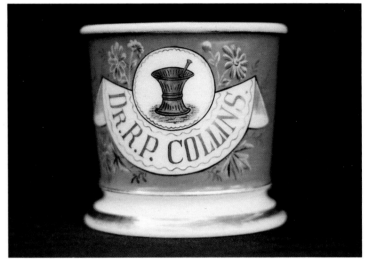

Doctor or druggist. *Courtesy of Dr. Ralph Nix.*

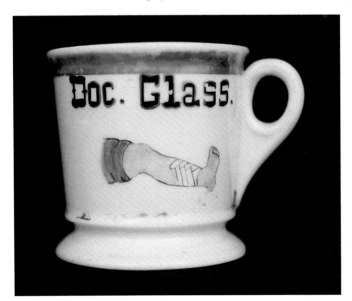

Doctor, bandaged leg. *Courtesy of Charles F. Kalb.*

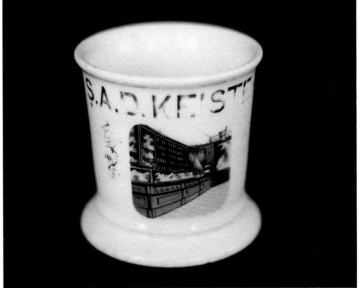

Pharmacist, interior view of pharmacy, rare. *Courtesy of Bernard Lukco.*

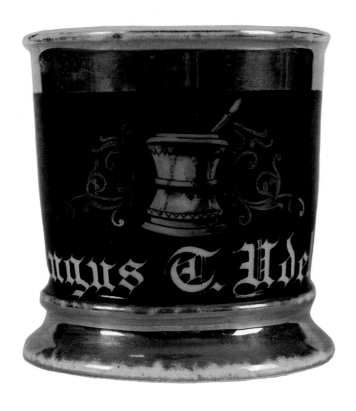

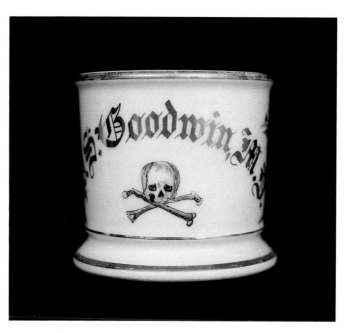

Pharmacist, mortar and pestle, black wrap. *Courtesy of Morris Pickerell, Jr.*

Doctor, skull and crossbones. *Courtesy of Charles F. Kalb.*

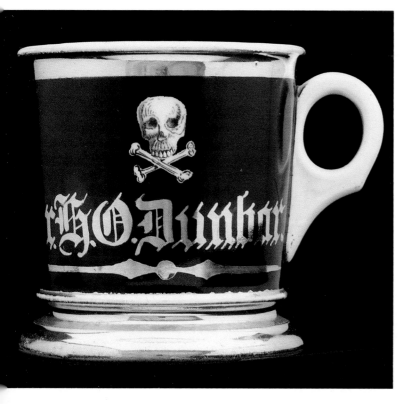

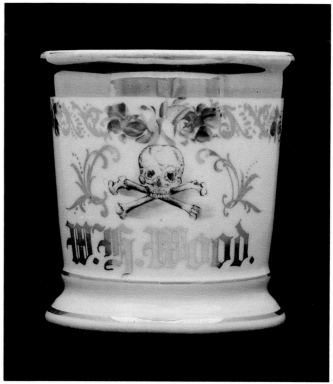

Doctor, skull and cross bones, black wrap. *Courtesy of Anthony Gugliotti.*

Pharmacist, Hamden, Connecticut, fancy example. *Anonymous.*

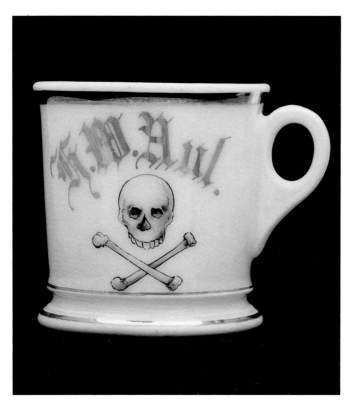

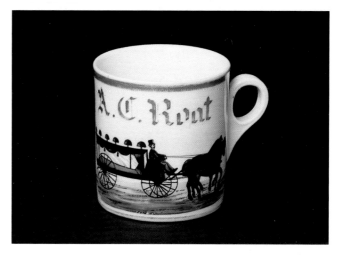

Hearse, undertaker. *Courtesy of Thomas and Penelope Nader.*

Pharmacist, skull and crossbones. The skull and crossbones design is used for doctor or pharmacist. It is not used for undertakers. *Anonymous.*

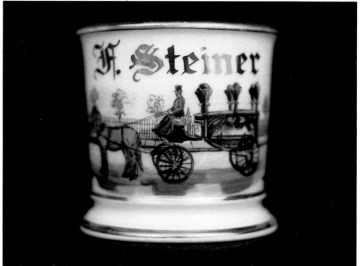

Hearse, undertaker. *Courtesy of Charles F. Kalb.*

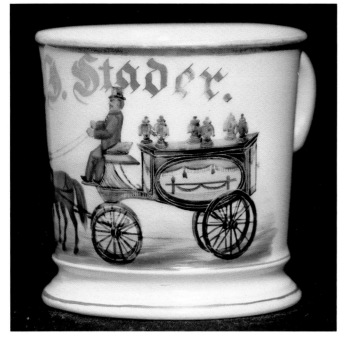

Hearse, undertaker. *Courtesy of Michael J. Griffin.*

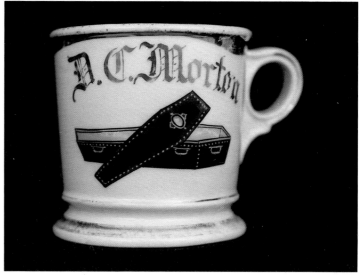

Coffin, undertaker or coffin maker. *Courtesy of Charles F. Kalb.*

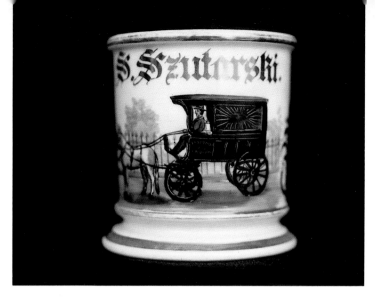

Dead wagon, brings remains to undertaker. *Courtesy of Charles F. Kalb.*

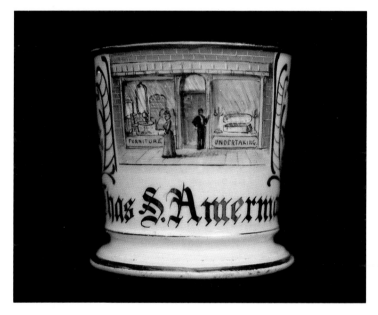

Undertaker and furniture store, rare. *Courtesy of Charles F. Kalb.*

Transportation

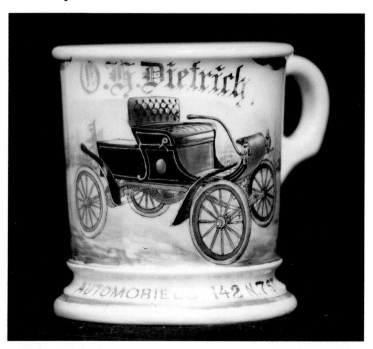

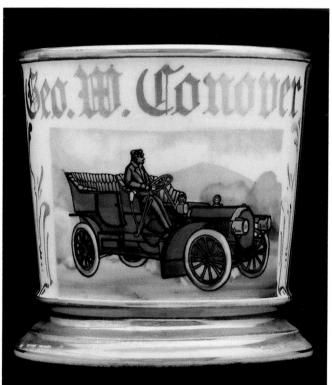

Auto, dealer's mug. *Courtesy of Michael J. Griffin.*

Early auto. *Courtesy of Anthony Gugliotti.*

Early auto, dealer's mug. *Courtesy of Michael J. Griffin.*

103

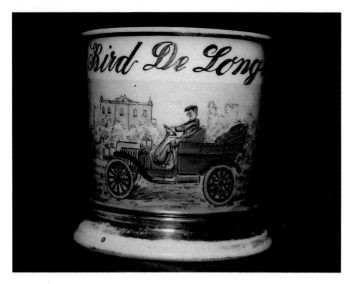

Early auto and driver, industrial build. *Courtesy of Raymond and Theresa Jones.*

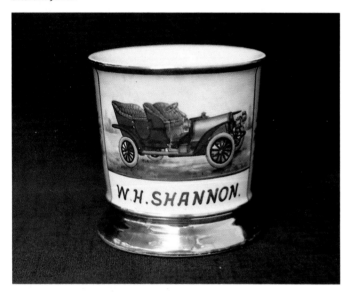

Early auto. *Courtesy of Bernard Lukco.*

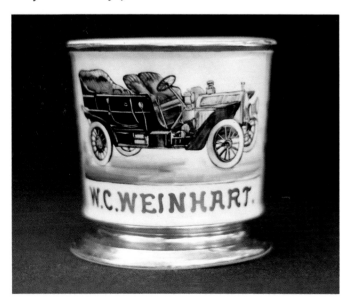

Early auto. *Courtesy of Dr. Ralph Nix.*

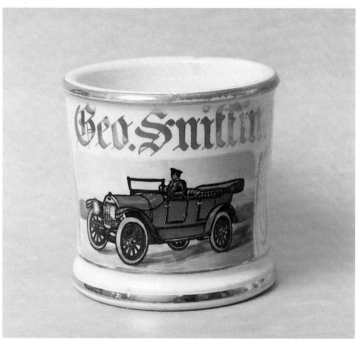

Auto with chauffeur. *Courtesy of David Giese.*

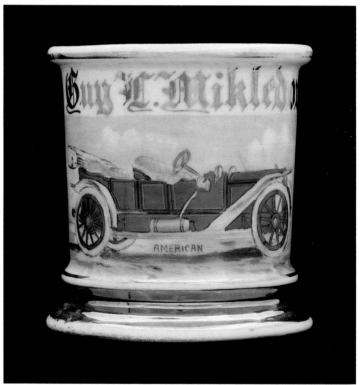

Auto, American Underslung, rare. *Anonymous.*

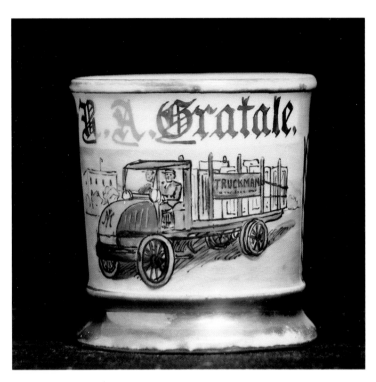

Early Mack truck. *Courtesy of Michael J. Griffin.*

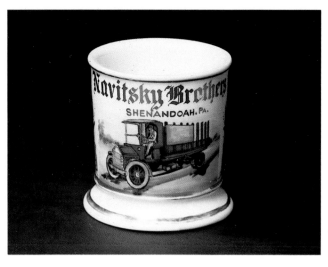

Truck, Shenandoah, Pennsylvania. *Courtesy of Thomas and Penelope Nader.*

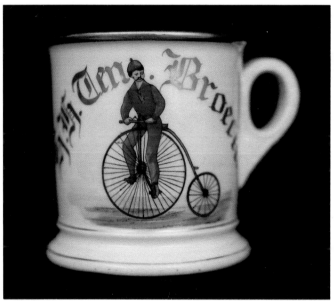

High wheel bicycle. *Courtesy of Charles F. Kalb.*

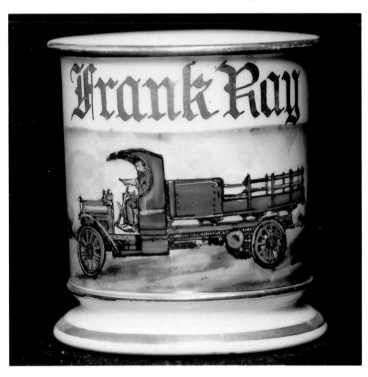

Truck. *Courtesy of Michael J. Griffin.*

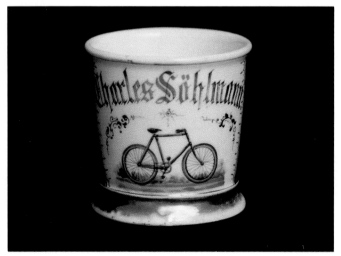

Bicycle. *Courtesy of Roland F. Porter.*

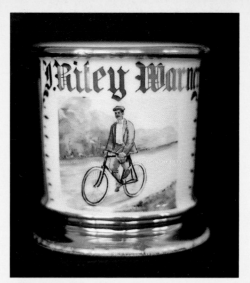

Bicycle with rider. *Courtesy of Bernard Lukco.*

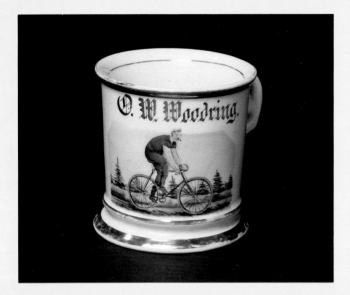

Bicycle with rider. *Courtesy of Thomas and Penelope Nader.*

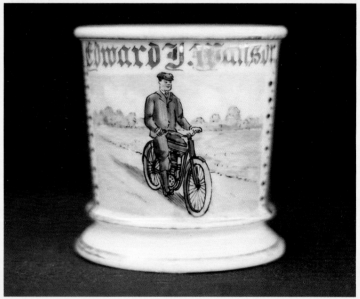

Motorcycle. *Courtesy of Dr. Ralph Nix.*

The Trolley

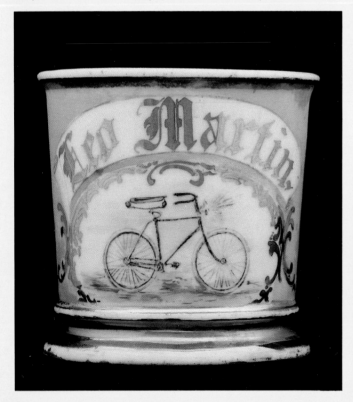

Bicycle with a light, messenger. *Courtesy of Anthony Gugliotti.*

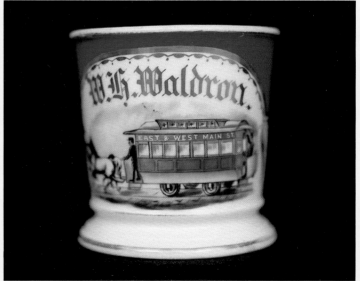

Horse-drawn trolley. *Courtesy of Charles F. Kalb.*

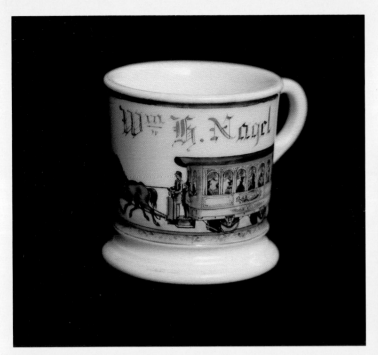

Horse-drawn trolley. *Courtesy of Roland F. Porter.*

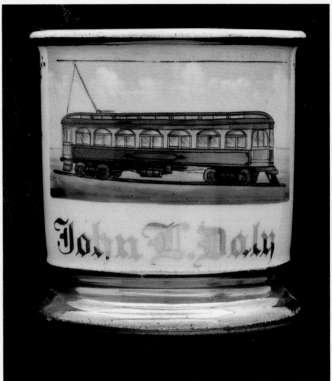

Electric trolley. *Anonymous.*

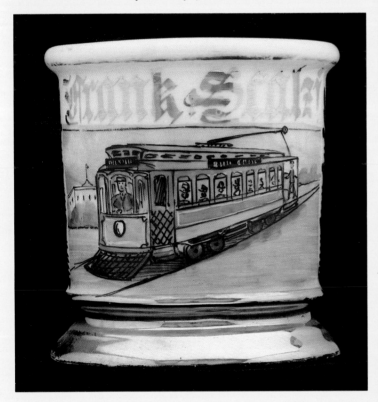

Electric trolley. *Courtesy of Anthony Gugliotti.*

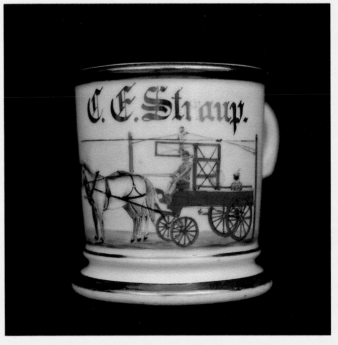

Electric trolley line repair wagon. *Courtesy of Charles F. Kalb.*

Four wheel locomotive. *Courtesy
of Morris Pickerell, Jr.*

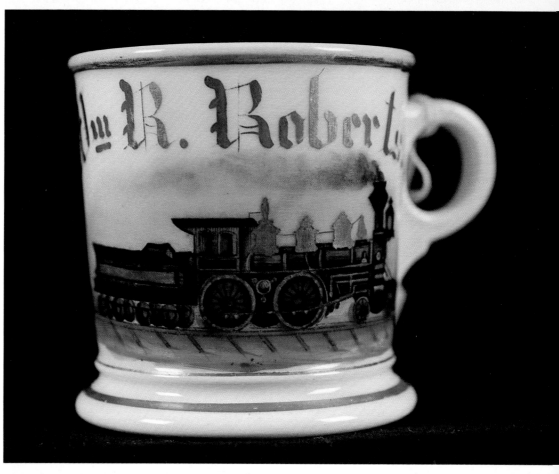

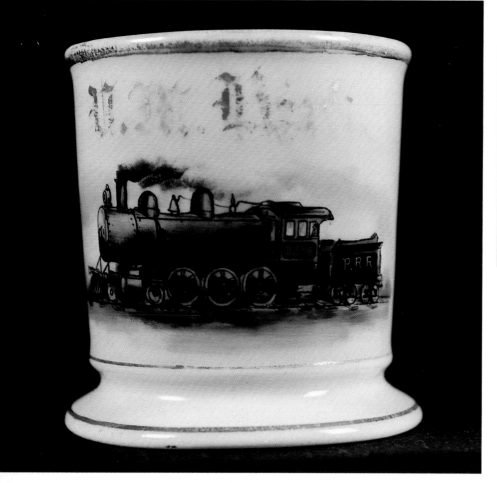

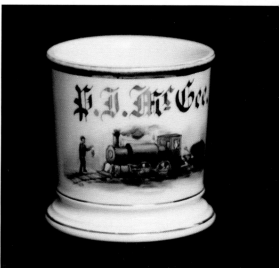

Locomotive with switchman. *Courtesy of
Roland F. Porter.*

Six wheel locomotive. *Courtesy of Morris
Pickerell, Jr.*

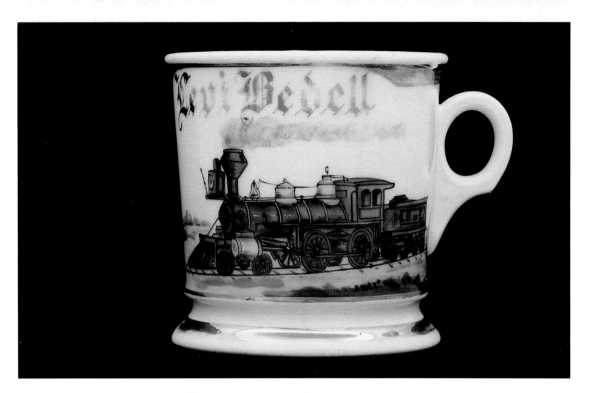

Locomotive, engineer's mug. *Anonymous.*

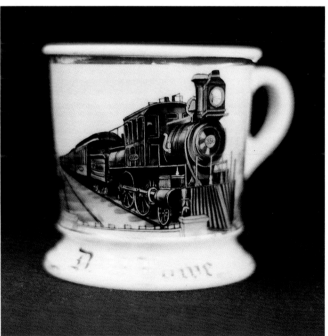

Camelback locomotive with cars. *Courtesy of Dr. Ralph Nix.*

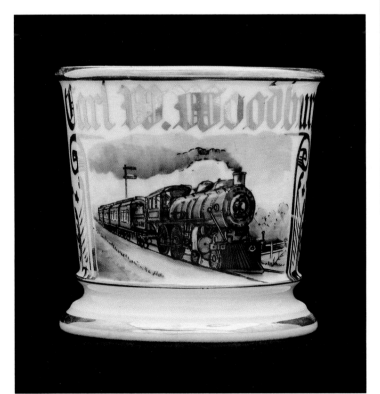

Locomotive with cars. *Anonymous.*

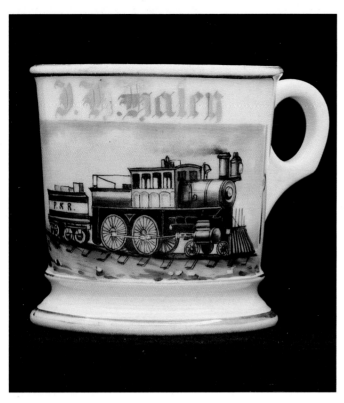

Camelback locomotive. *Anonymous.*

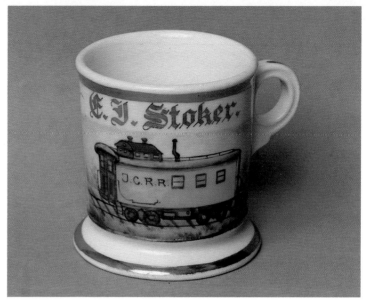

Caboose. *Courtesy of David Giese.*

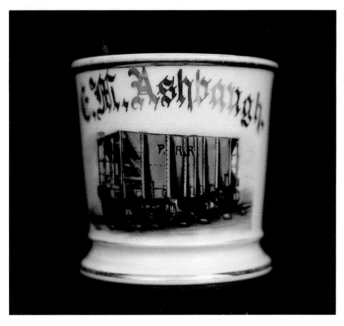

Coal car. *Courtesy of Charles F. Kalb.*

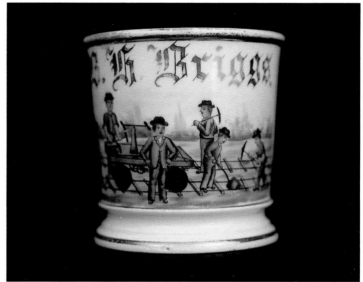

Section gang. *Courtesy of Charles F. Kalb.*

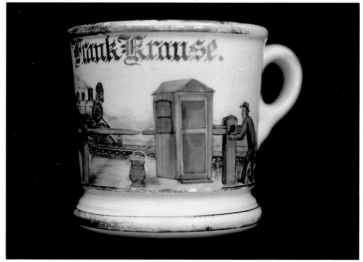

Crossing watchman. *Courtesy of Charles F. Kalb.*

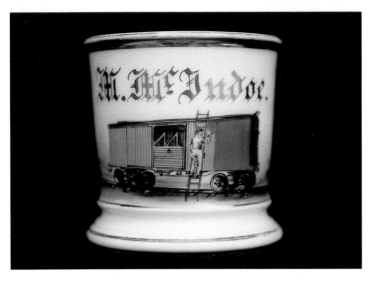

Yard painter, painting a boxcar. *Courtesy of Charles F. Kalb.*

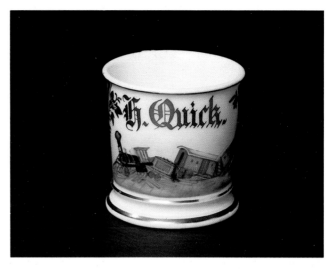

Train wreck, a wrecker's mug. *Courtesy of Thomas and Penelope Nader.*

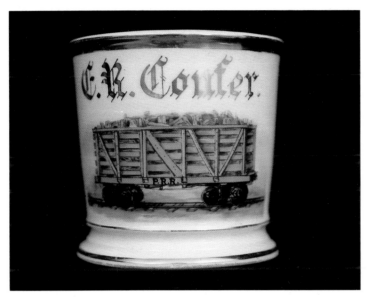

Metal ingot car. *Courtesy of Charles F. Kalb.*

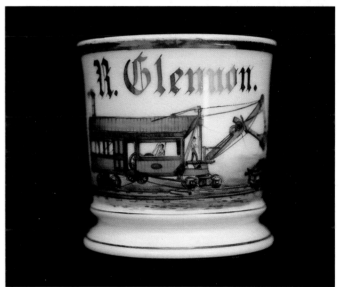

Railroad wrecker. *Courtesy of Charles F. Kalb.*

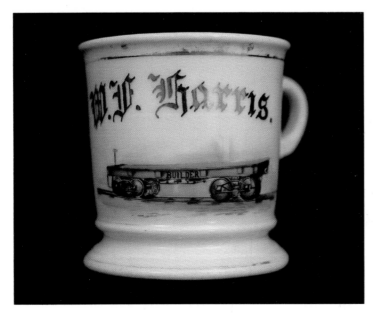

Flat car builder. *Courtesy of Charles F. Kalb.*

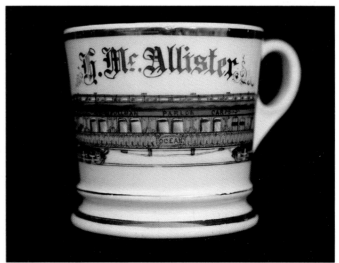

Private car, "Ocean." *Courtesy of Charles F. Kalb.*

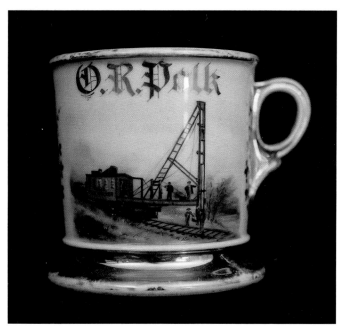

Railroad pile driver, rare. *Courtesy of Charles F. Kalb.*

News and Letters

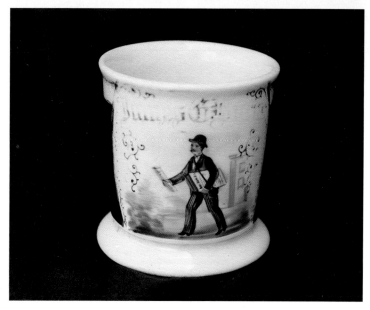

Newspaper man. *Courtesy of Bernard Lukco.*

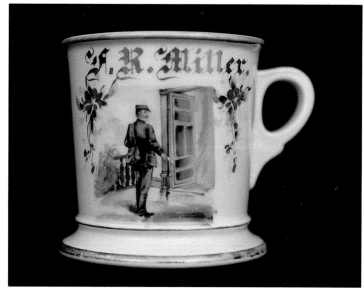

Postman at door. *Courtesy of Charles F. Kalb.*

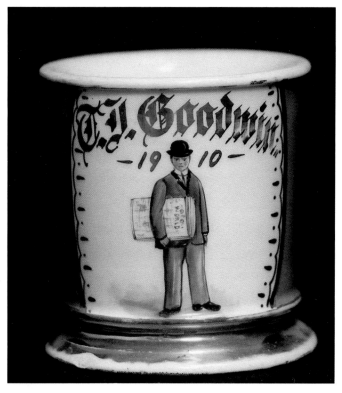

Newspaper man, the "World." *Courtesy of Michael J. Griffin.*

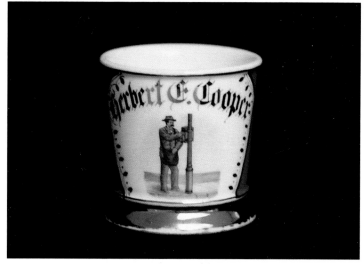

Postman at letter box. *Courtesy of Roland F. Porter.*

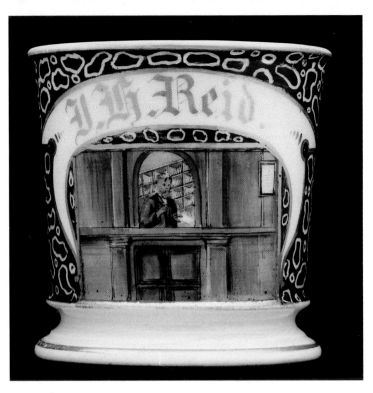

Post office, letter handler. *Courtesy of Anthony Gugliotti.*

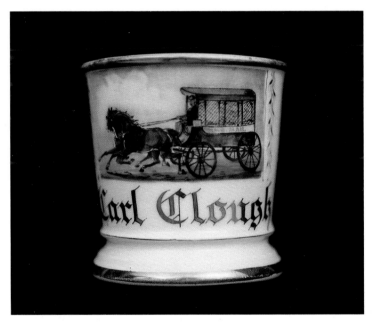

Rural mail wagon. *Courtesy of Charles F. Kalb.*

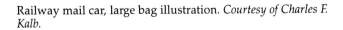

Railway mail car, large bag illustration. *Courtesy of Charles F. Kalb.*

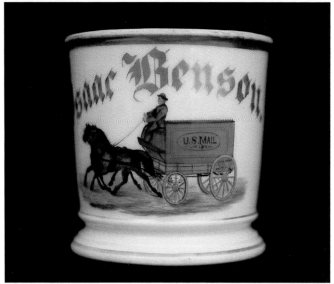

Bulk mail wagon. *Courtesy of Charles F. Kalb.*

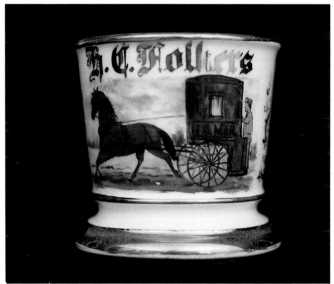

Special delivery wagon. *Courtesy of Charles F. Kalb.*

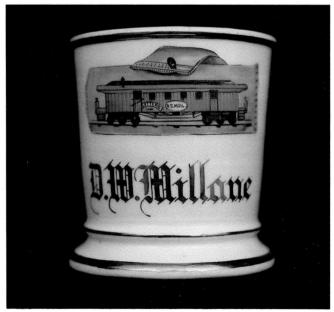

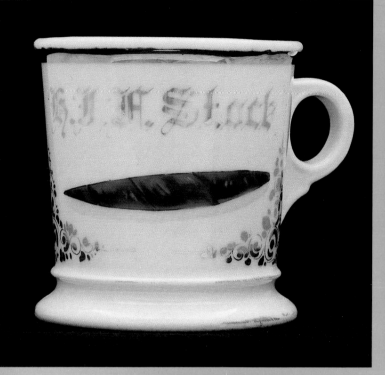

Cigar. *Anonymous.*

Bunch of cigars. *Courtesy of Dr. Ralph Nix.*

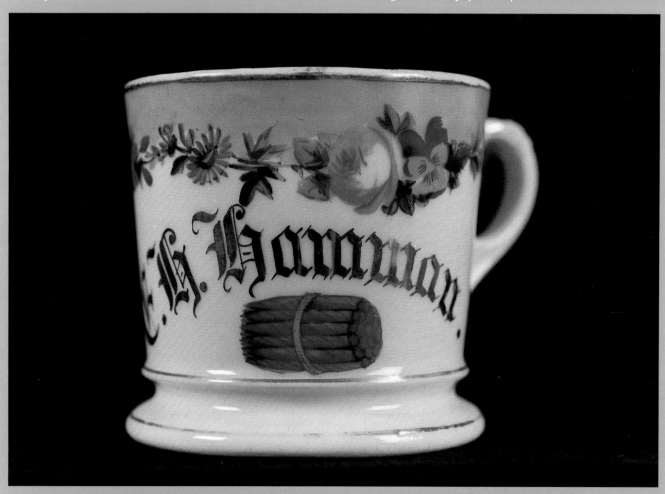

Bunch of cigars, fancy. *Courtesy of Morris Pickerell, Jr.*

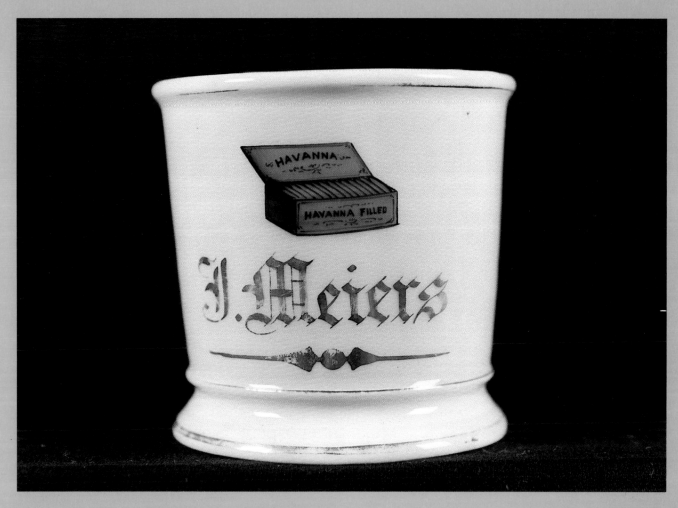

Box of cigars. *Courtesy of Morris Pickerell, Jr.*

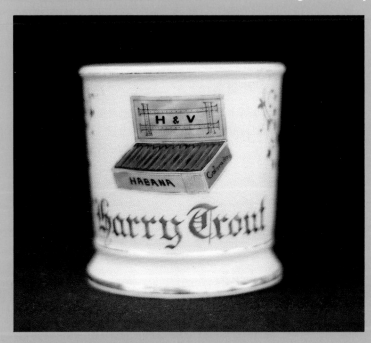

Box of cigars. *Courtesy of Dr. Ralph Nix.*

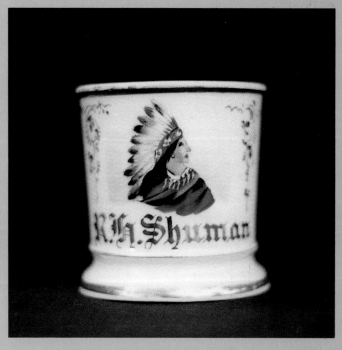

Indian, tobacco related. *Courtesy of Dr. Ralph Nix.*

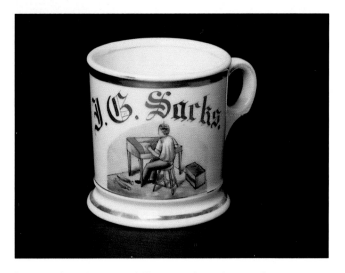

Cigar maker. *Courtesy of Thomas and Penelope Nader.*

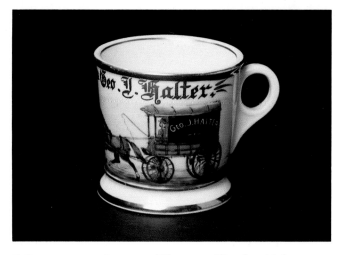

Delivery wagon. *Courtesy of Thomas and Penelope Nader.*

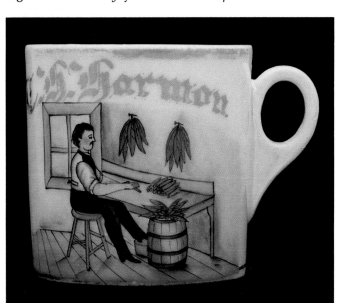

Cigar roller. *Anonymous.*

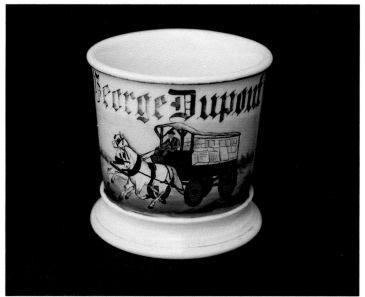

Delivery wagon. *Courtesy of Bernard Lukco.*

Coal delivery wagon. *Courtesy of David Giese.*

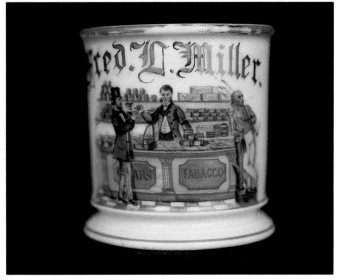

Tobacco store with wooden Indian. *Courtesy of Charles F. Kalb.*

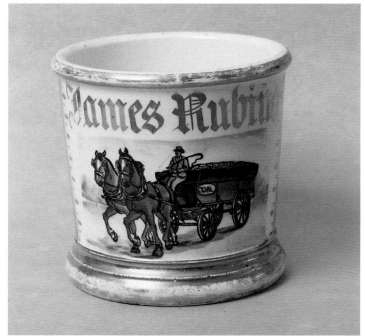

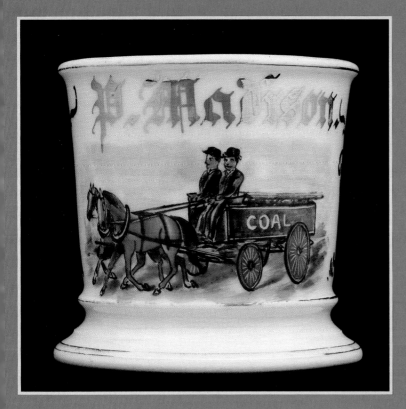

Coal delivery wagon. *Courtesy of Anthony Gugliotti.*

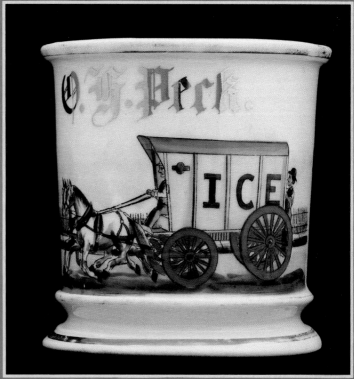

Ice wagon. *Courtesy of Anthony Gugliotti.*

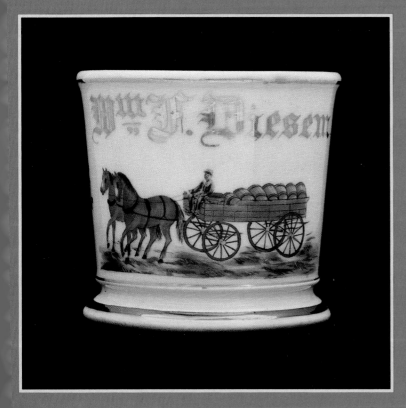

Barrel wagon. *Anonymous.*

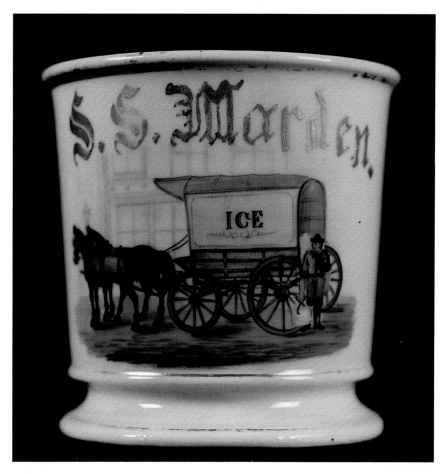

Ice wagon. *Courtesy of Morris Pickerell, Jr.*

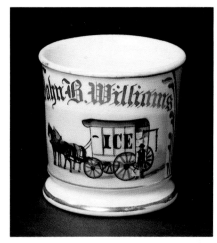

Ice wagon. *Courtesy of Thomas and Penelope Nader.*

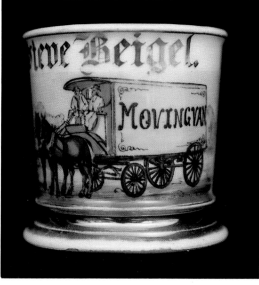

Moving van. *Courtesy of Charles F. Kalb.*

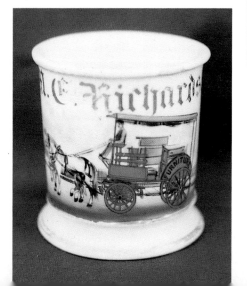

Furniture delivery wagon. *Courtesy of Bernard Lukco.*

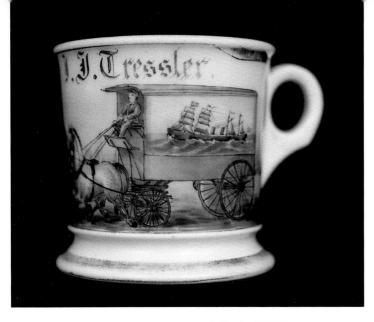

Ship's chandler wagon. *Courtesy of Charles F. Kalb.*

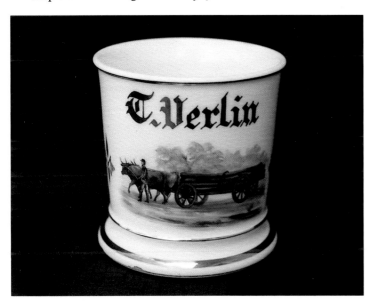

Ox drawn logging wagon. *Courtesy of Bernard Lukco.*

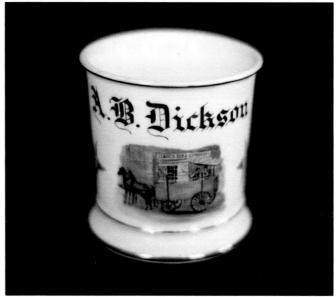

Lumber wagon. *Courtesy of Bernard Lukco.*

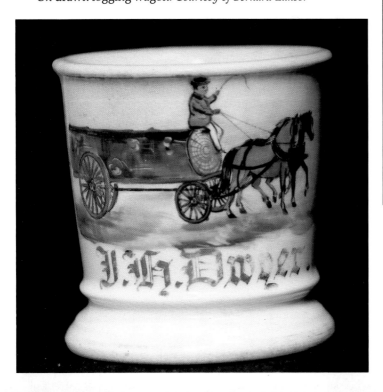

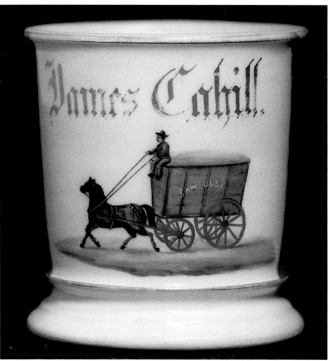

Saw dust wagon. *Courtesy of Michael J. Griffin.*

Logging wagon, one huge log. *Courtesy of Michael J. Griffin.*

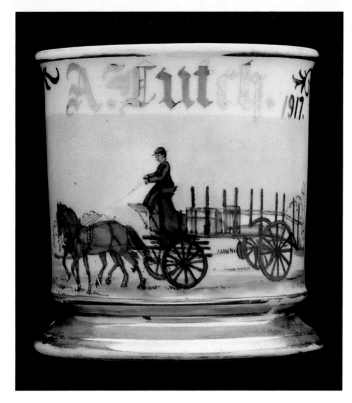

Stake wagon. *Courtesy of Anthony Gugliotti.*

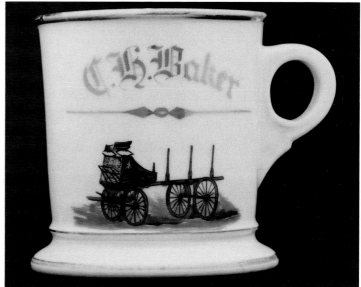

Wagon salesman. *Courtesy of Anthony Gugliotti.*

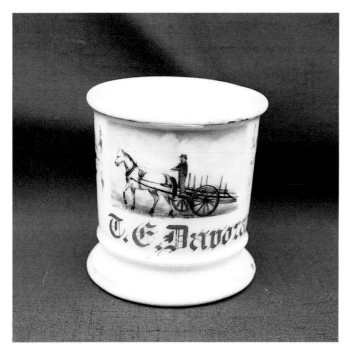

Stake wagon. *Courtesy of Bernard Lukco.*

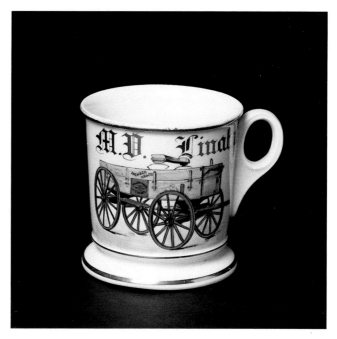

Wagon maker, Jackson Wagons. *Courtesy of Thomas and Penelope Nader.*

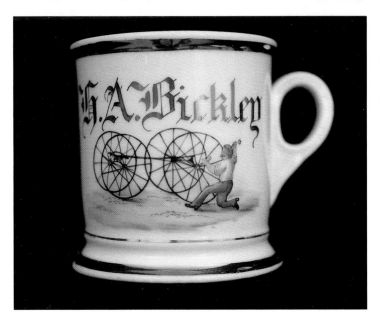

Buggy maker. *Courtesy of Charles F. Kalb.*

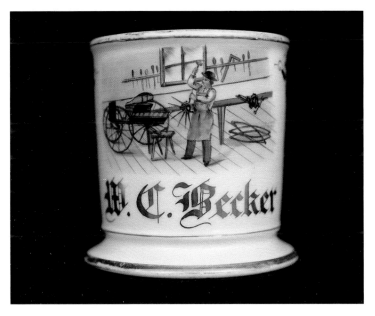

Wheelwright. *Courtesy of Charles F. Kalb.*

Wagon wheel, wheelwright. *Courtesy of Bernard Lukco.*

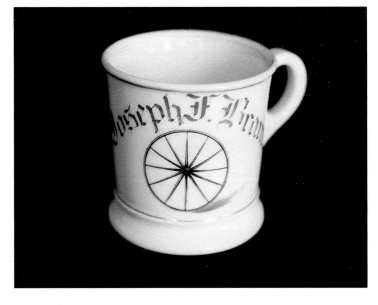

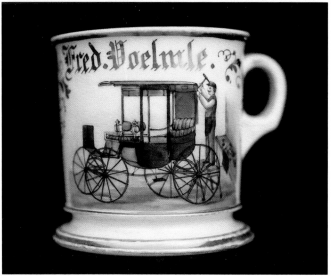

Carriage trimmer. *Courtesy of Charles F. Kalb.*

Men at Work

Men of Stone

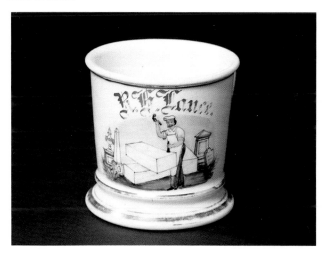

Monument cutter. *Courtesy of Thomas and Penelope Nader.*

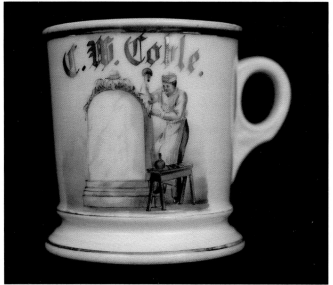

Tombstone cutter. *Courtesy of Charles F. Kalb.*

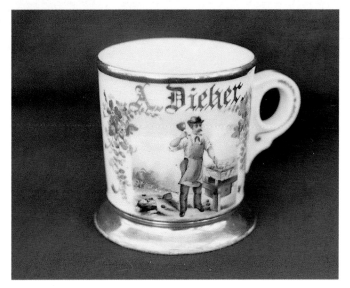

Stone cutter. *Courtesy of Bernard Lukco.*

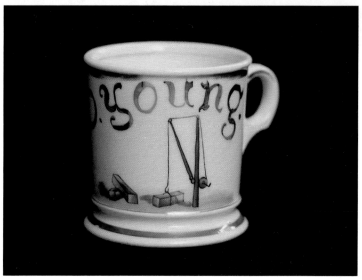

Winch. *Courtesy of Roland F. Porter.*

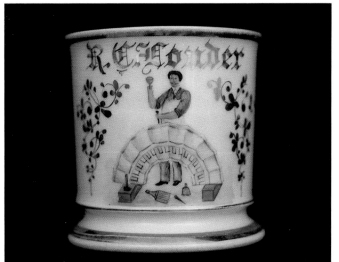

Marble arch cutter. *Courtesy of Charles F. Kalb.*

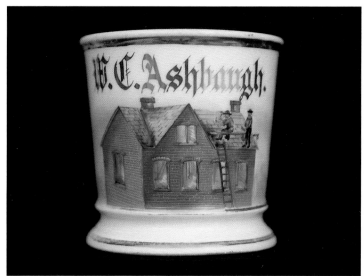

Slate roofers. *Courtesy of Charles F. Kalb.*

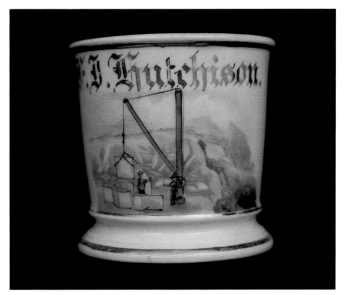

Marble quarry with winch. *Courtesy of Charles F. Kalb.*

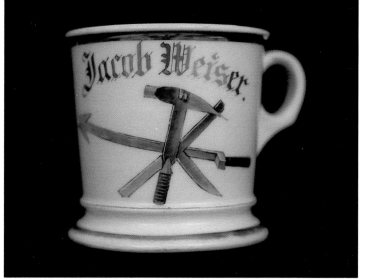

Slate roofer's tools. *Courtesy of Charles F. Kalb.*

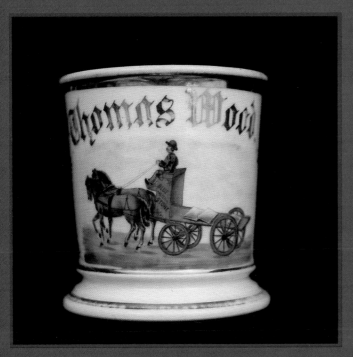

"Blue Stone" slate wagon. *Courtesy of Charles F. Kalb.*

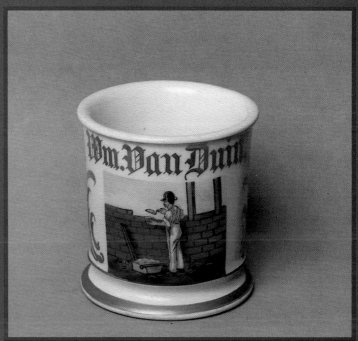

Brick mason. *Courtesy of David Giese.*

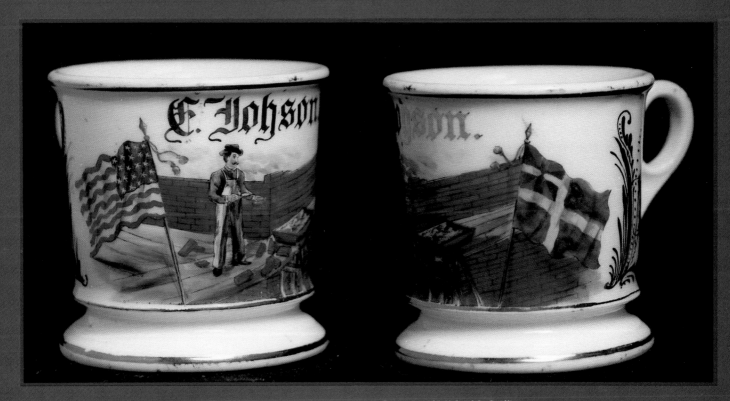

Swedish American brick mason. *Courtesy of Michael J. Griffin.*

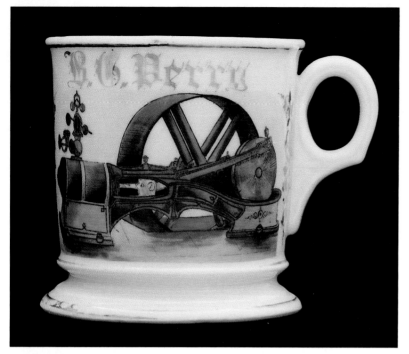

Stationary engine. *Anonymous.*

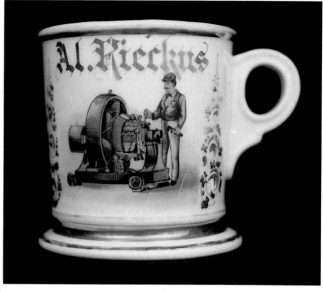

Man working on Dynamo. *Courtesy of Charles F. Kalb.*

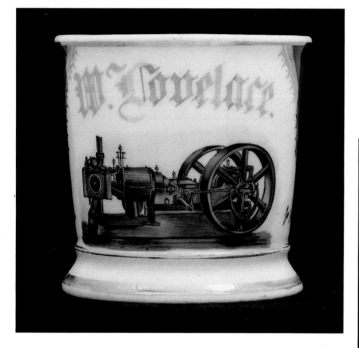

Stationary engine. *Anonymous.*

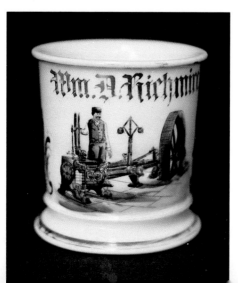

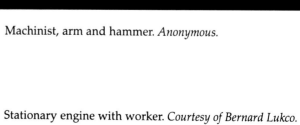

Machinist, arm and hammer. *Anonymous.*

Stationary engine with worker. *Courtesy of Bernard Lukco.*

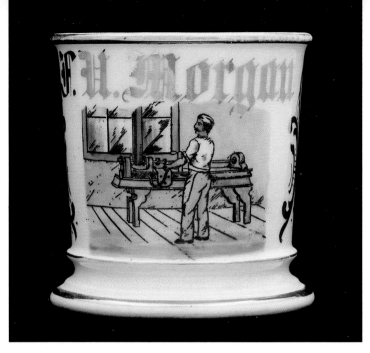

Machinist, man at lathe. *Anonymous.*

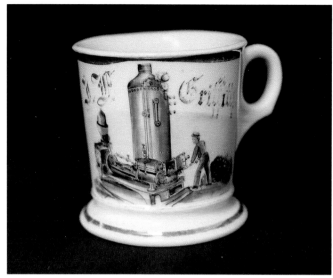

Boiler stoker. *Courtesy of Bernard Lukco.*

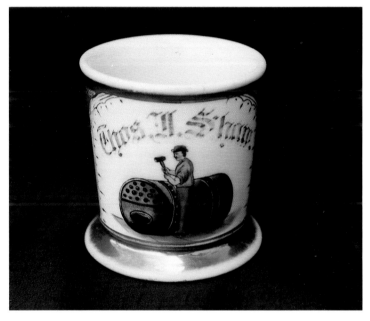

Boiler maker. *Courtesy of Bernard Lukco.*

Boiler maker, two men. *Courtesy of Charles F. Kalb.*

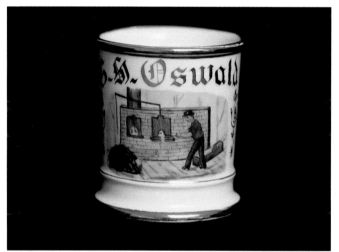

Kiln or furnace worker. *Courtesy of Roland F. Porter.*

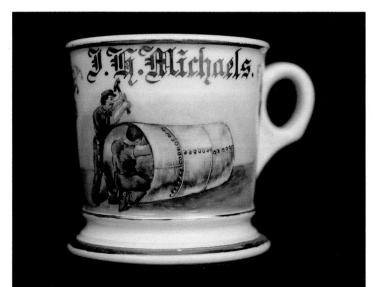

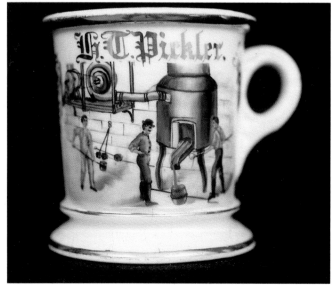

Steel converter. *Courtesy of Charles F. Kalb.*

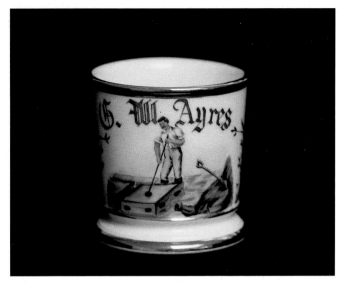

Iron puddler. *Courtesy of Roland F. Porter.*

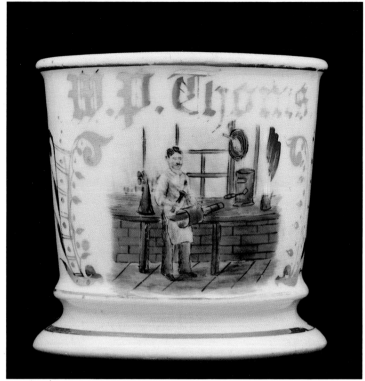

Tinsmith. *Courtesy of Anthony Gugliotti.*

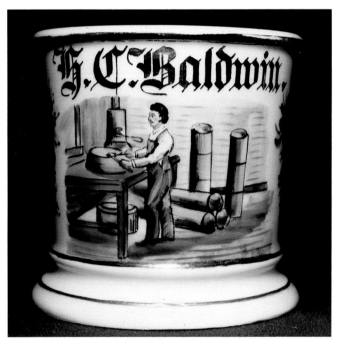

Tinsmith. *Courtesy of Raymond and Theresa Jones.*

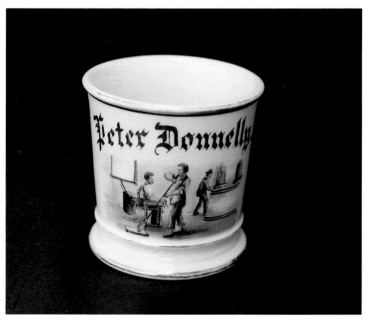

Glassblower. *Courtesy of Bernard Lukco.*

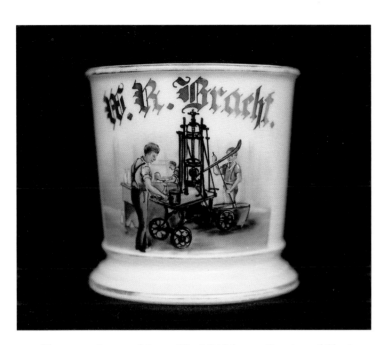

Glass pressing machine, with child laborer. *Courtesy of Charles F. Kalb.*

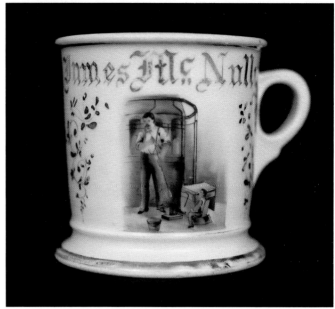

Glassblower with child laborer or apprentice. *Courtesy of Charles F. Kalb.*

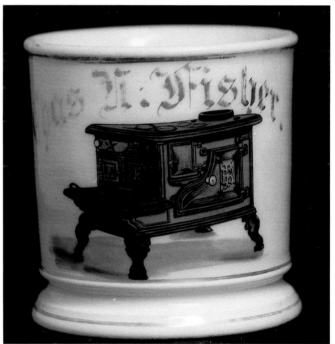

Manufacturer, Fisher Stoves. *Courtesy of Michael J. Griffin.*

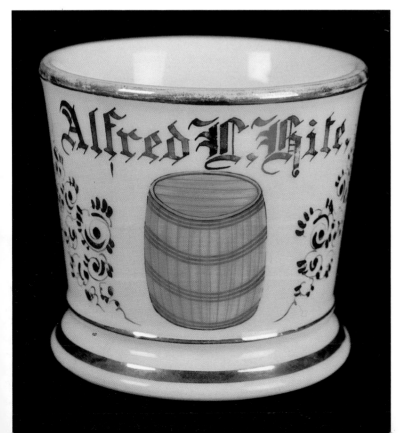

Cooper, barrel maker. *Courtesy of Morris Pickerell, Jr.*

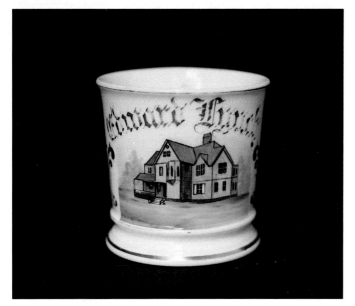

House builder. *Courtesy of Bernard Lukco.*

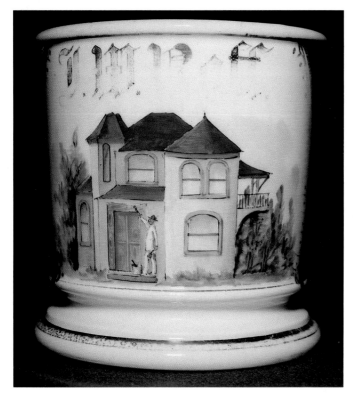

House painter. *Courtesy of Raymond and Theresa Jones.*

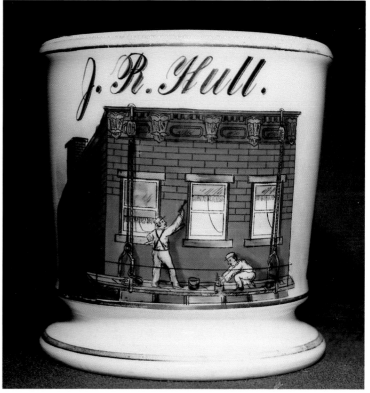

Painters, brick building. *Courtesy of Raymond and Theresa Jones.*

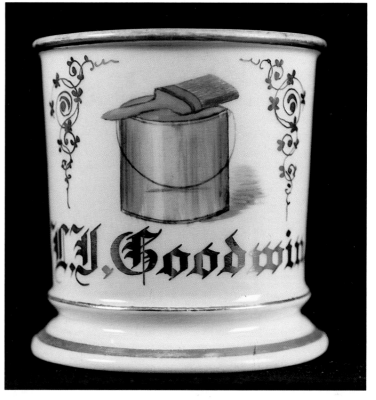

Painter, bucket and brush. *Courtesy of Morris Pickerell, Jr.*

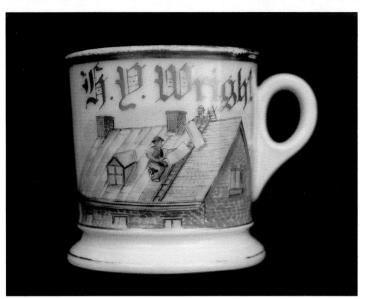

Tin roofers. *Courtesy of Charles F. Kalb.*

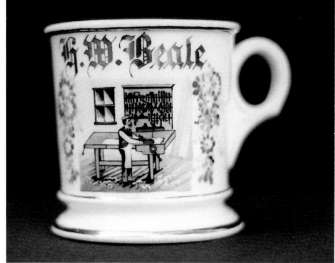

Cabinet maker or carpenter. *Courtesy of Dr. Ralph Nix.*

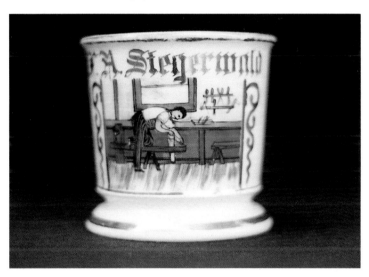

Carpenter. *Courtesy of Dr. Ralph Nix.*

Carpenter's tools. *Courtesy of Anthony Gugliotti.*

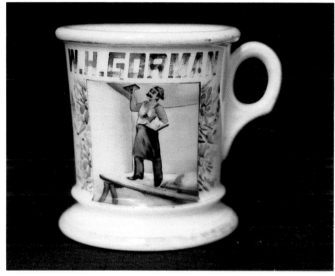

Plasterer. *Courtesy of Bernard Lukco.*

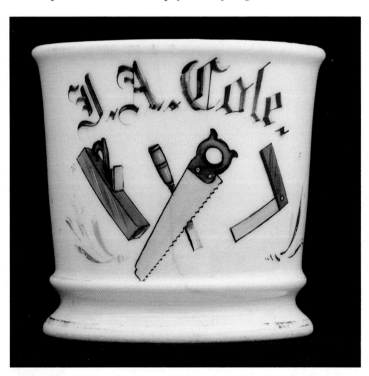

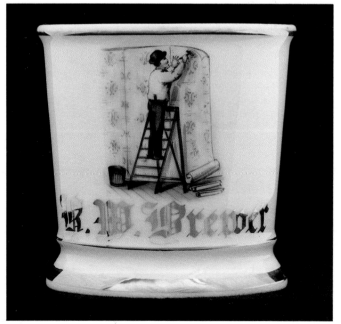

Wall paper hanger. *Anonymous.*

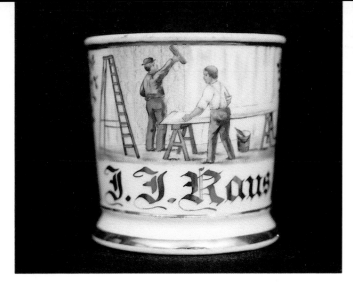

Wall paper hangers. *Anonymous.*

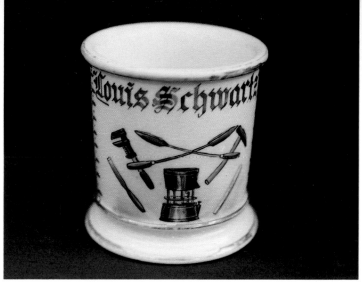

Plumber tools. *Courtesy of Bernard Lukco.*

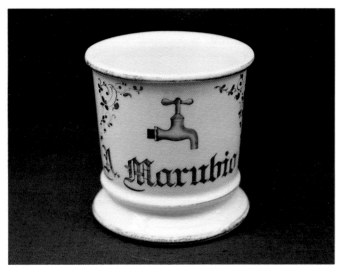

Plumber or pipe fitter. *Courtesy of Bernard Lukco.*

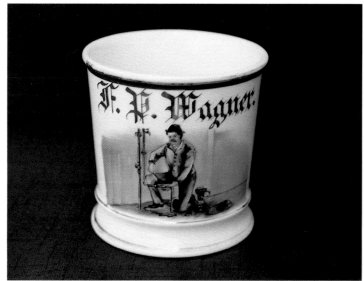

Working plumber. *Courtesy of Bernard Lukco.*

Working plumber. *Courtesy of Anthony Gugliotti.*

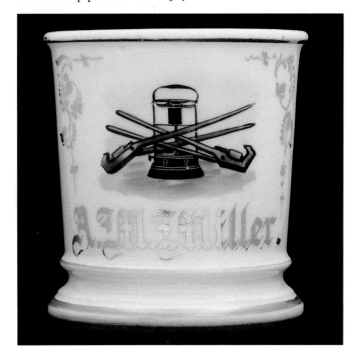

Plumber tools. *Anonymous.*

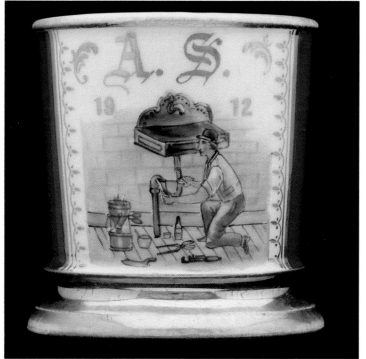

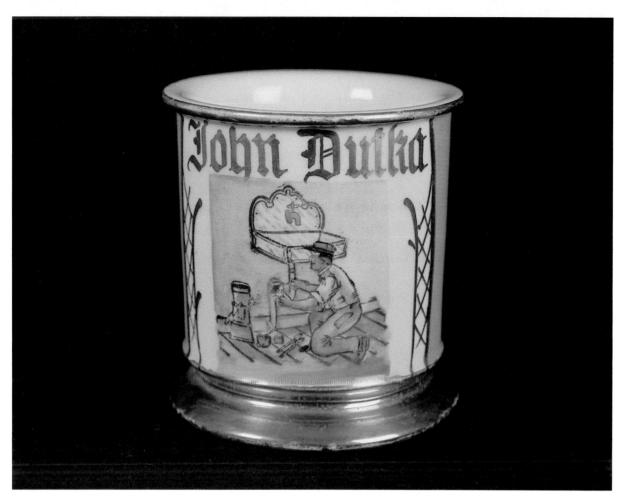

Working plumber. *Courtesy of Morris Pickerell, Jr.*

Outside Work

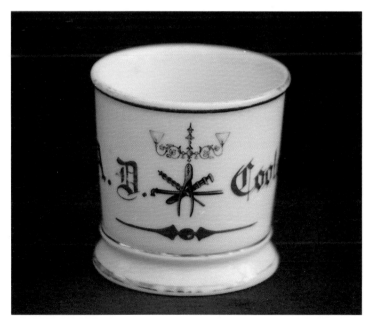

Gas pipe fitter. *Courtesy of Bernard Lukco.*

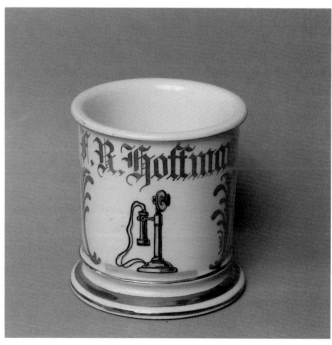

Candlestick phone, telephone related. *Courtesy of David Giese.*

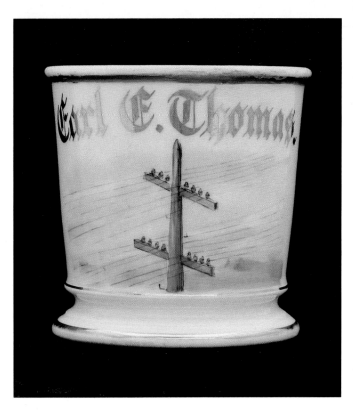

Telephone lineman. *Anonymous.*

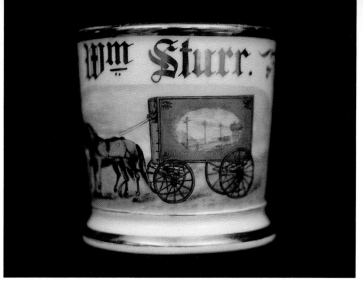

Telephone lineman's wagon. *Courtesy of Charles F. Kalb.*

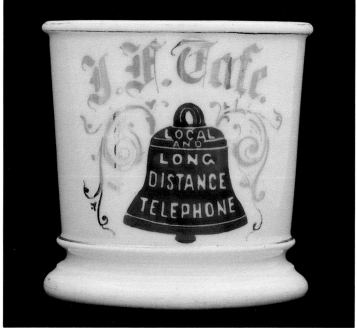

Telephone company foreman. *Anonymous.*

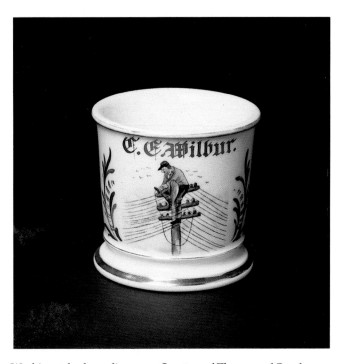

Working telephone lineman. *Courtesy of Thomas and Penelope Nader.*

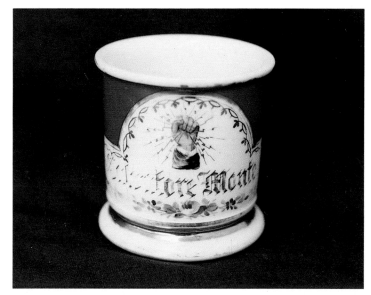

Electrician. *Courtesy of Bernard Lukco.*

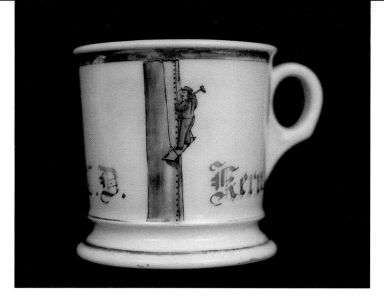

Steeple jack. *Courtesy of Charles F. Kalb.*

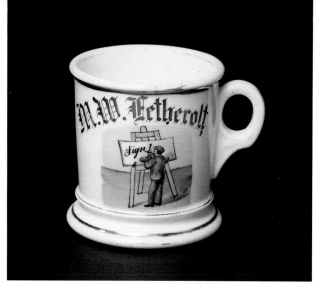

Sign painter. *Courtesy of Thomas and Penelope Nader.*

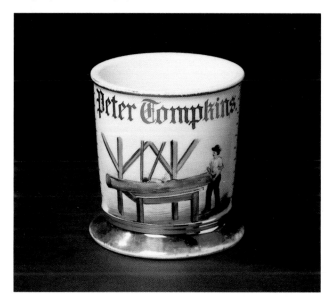

Saw mill operator. *Courtesy of Thomas and Penelope Nader.*

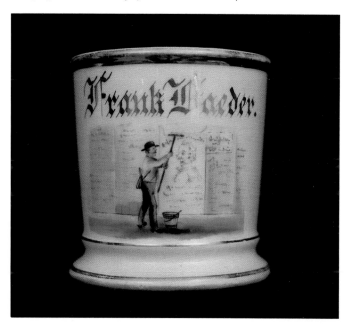

Poster hanger. *Courtesy of Charles F. Kalb.*

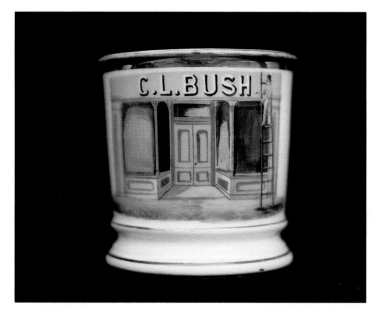

Sign painter. *Courtesy of Charles F. Kalb.*

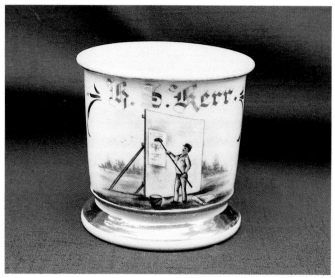

Poster hanger. *Courtesy of Bernard Lukco.*

133

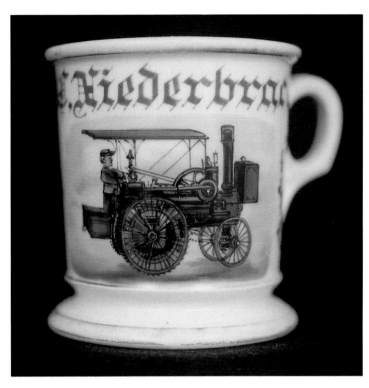

Tractor operator. *Courtesy of Charles F. Kalb.*

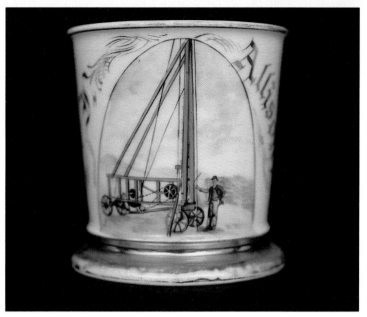

Water well driller. *Courtesy of Charles F. Kalb.*

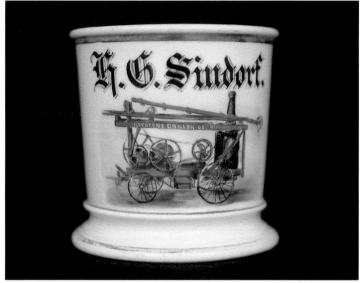

Steam water well driller. *Courtesy of Charles F. Kalb.*

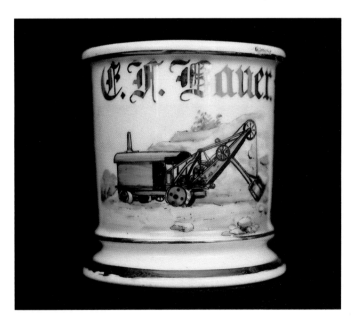

Steam shovel operator. *Courtesy of Charles F. Kalb.*

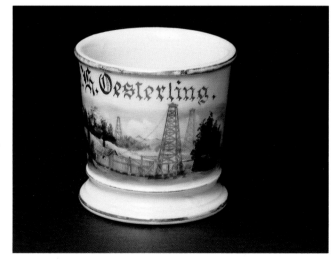

Oil well worker. *Courtesy of Thomas and Penelope Nader.*

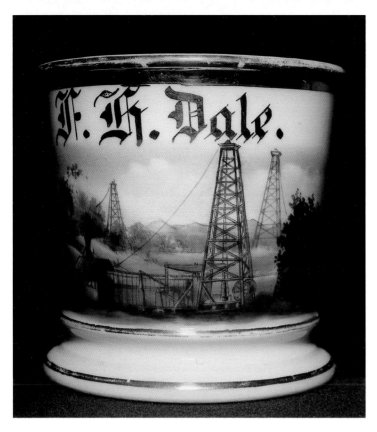

Standard oil company tanker wagon, rare. *Courtesy of Charles F. Kalb.*

Oil well worker. *Courtesy of Raymond and Theresa Jones.*

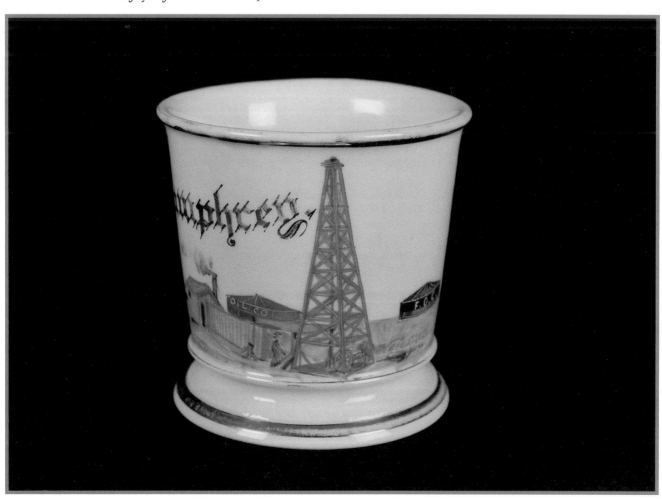

Oil well and tank farm. *Courtesy of Morris Pickerell, Jr.*

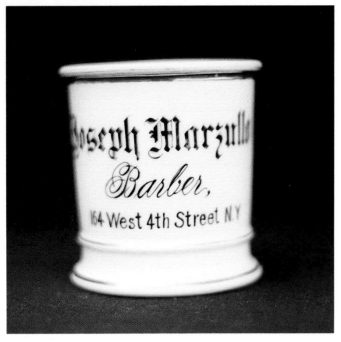

Barber, occupational by courtesy. *Courtesy of Dr. Ralph Nix.*

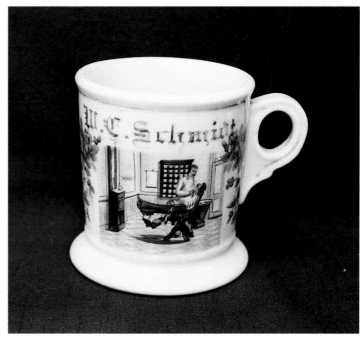

Working barber. *Courtesy of Bernard Lukco.*

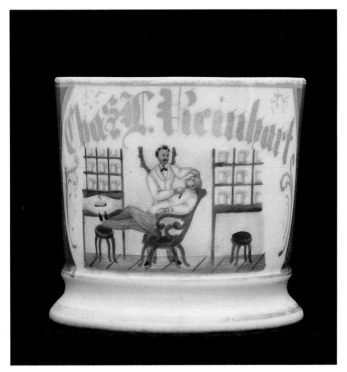

Working barber. *Anonymous.*

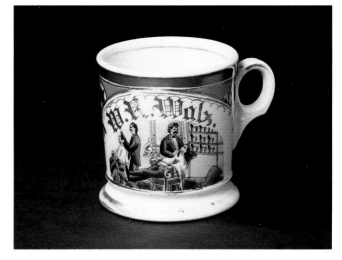

Barber shop. *Courtesy of Thomas and Penelope Nader.*

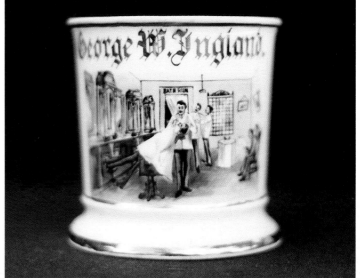

Barber shop, bathroom, customers, with lots of detail. *Courtesy of Dr. Ralph Nix.*

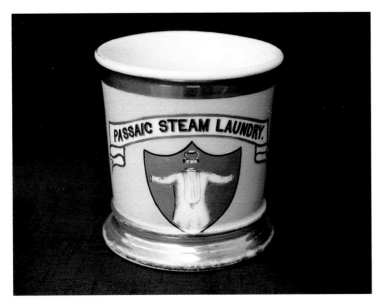

Laundry owner. *Courtesy of Bernard Lukco.*

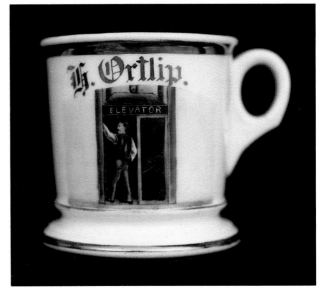

Elevator operator. *Courtesy of Charles F. Kalb.*

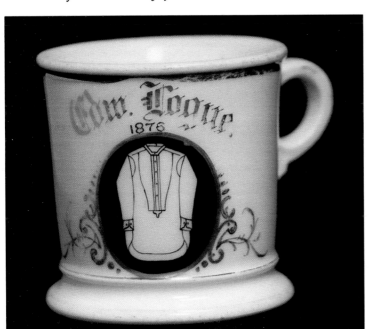

Laundry worker or owner. *Courtesy of Michael J. Griffin.*

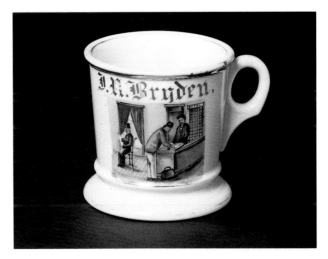

Hotel desk clerk. *Courtesy of Thomas and Penelope Nader.*

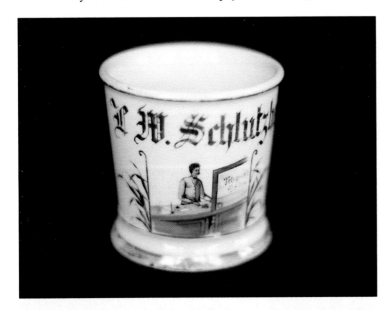

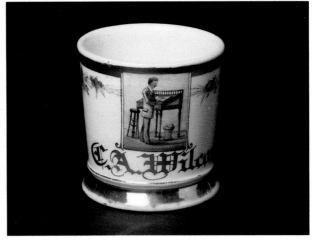

Clerk. *Courtesy of Thomas and Penelope Nader.*

Telegraph operator. *Courtesy of Bernard Lukco.*

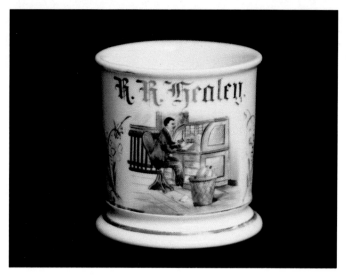

Executive at roll top desk. *Courtesy of Roland F. Porter.*

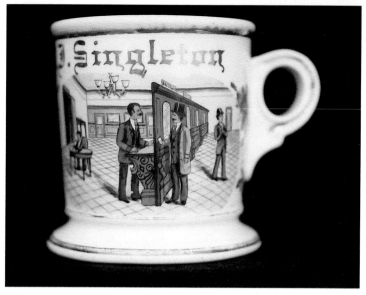

Bank teller. *Courtesy of Charles F. Kalb.*

Sales

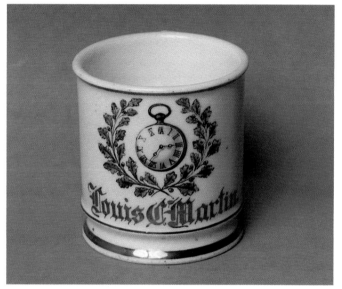

Pocket watch, jeweler. *Courtesy of David Giese.*

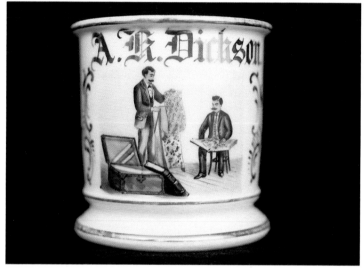

Wall paper salesman. *Courtesy of Charles F. Kalb.*

Watch and clock store, sales. *Courtesy of Charles F. Kalb.*

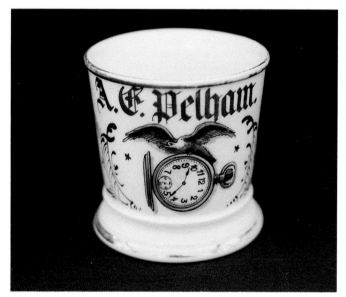

Pocket watch with eagle, jeweler. *Courtesy of Bernard Lukco.*

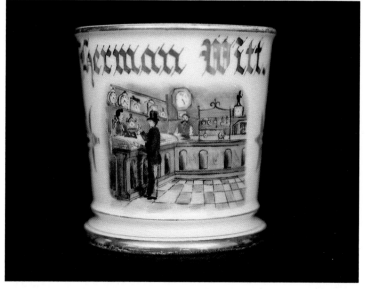

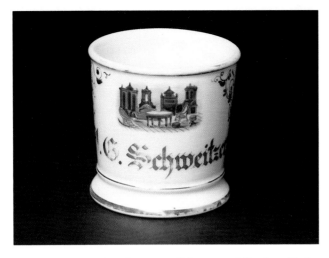

Furniture store, sales. *Courtesy of Thomas and Penelope Nader.*

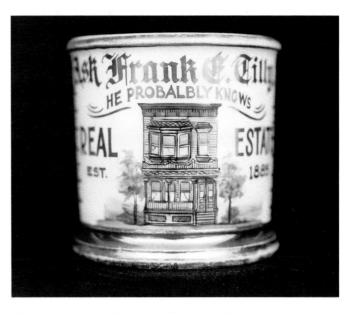

Real estate sales. *Courtesy of Charles F. Kalb.*

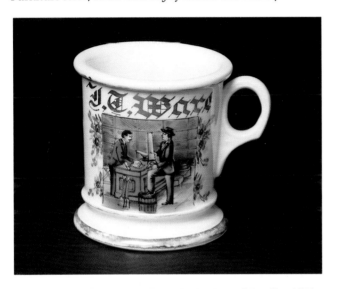

Hardware store, sales. *Courtesy of Thomas and Penelope Nader.*

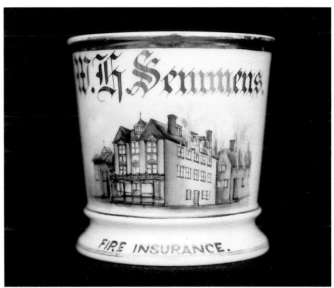

Fire insurance salesman. *Courtesy of Charles F. Kalb.*

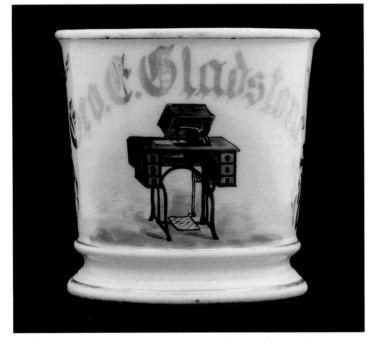

Sewing machine salesman. *Anonymous.*

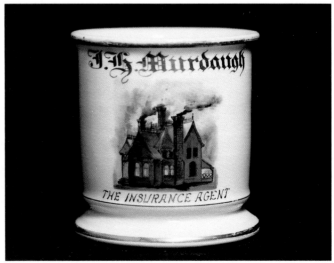

Insurance agent. *Courtesy of Michael J. Griffin.*

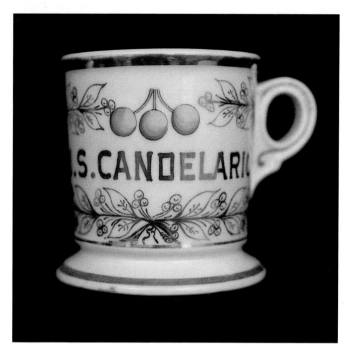

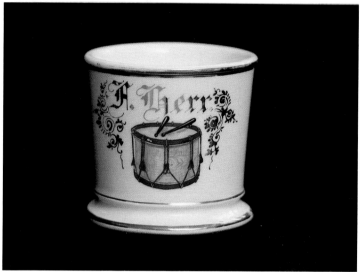

Pawn broker. *Courtesy of Charles F. Kalb.*

Drum. *Courtesy of Roland F. Porter.*

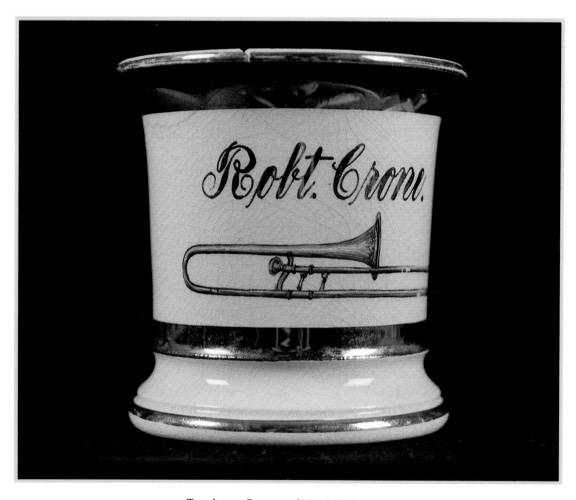

Trombone. *Courtesy of Morris Pickerell, Jr.*

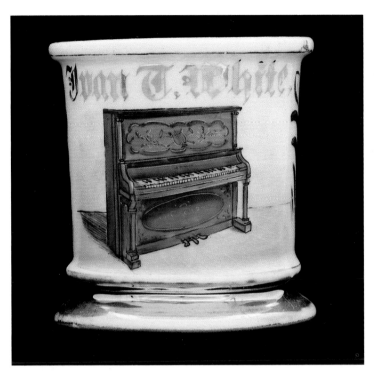

Piano, Hartford band leader. *Anonymous.*

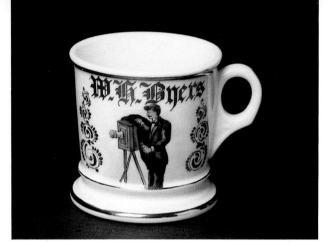

Photographer. *Courtesy of Thomas and Penelope Nader.*

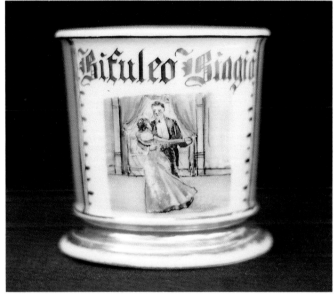

Dance instructor. *Courtesy of Dr. Ralph Nix.*

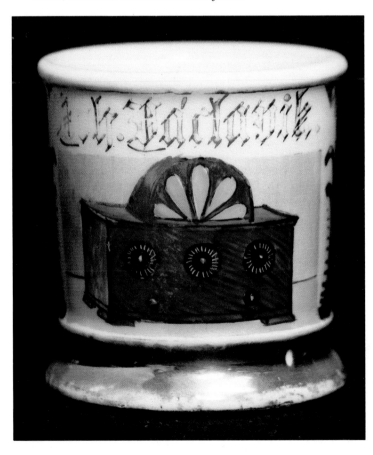

Radio, salesman. *Courtesy of Michael J. Griffin.*

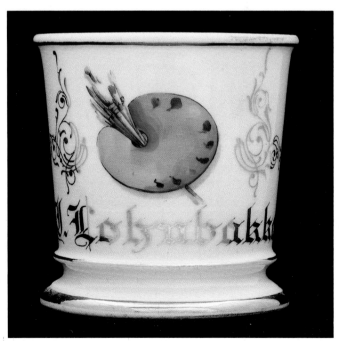

Artist, pallet. *Anonymous.*

Photographic

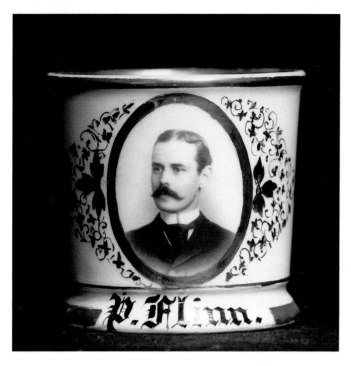

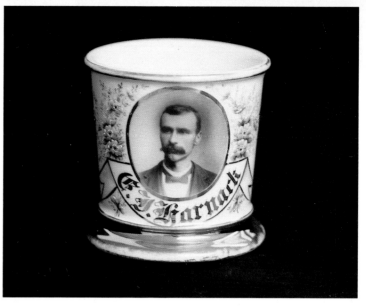

Personalized cameo. *Courtesy of Roland F. Porter.*

Personalized cameo. *Courtesy of Michael J. Griffin.*

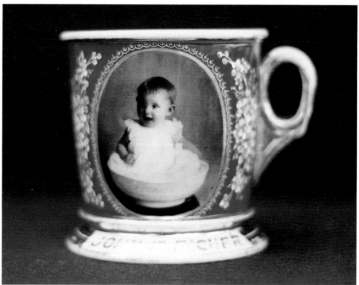

Personalized cameo, owner's baby. *Courtesy of Dr. Ralph Nix.*

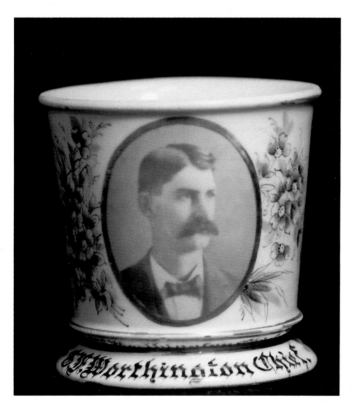

Personalized cameo, the "chief". *Courtesy of Michael J. Griffin.*

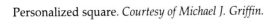

Personalized square. *Courtesy of Michael J. Griffin.*

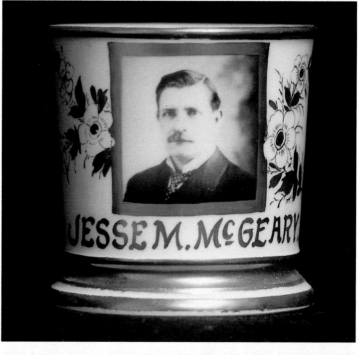

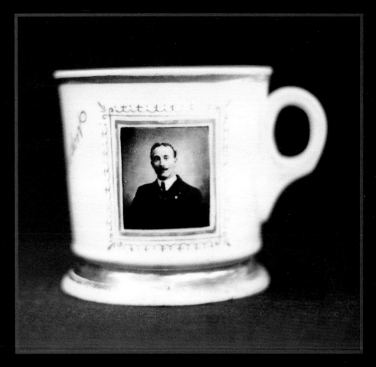

Non-personalized square. *Courtesy of Dr. Ralph Nix.*

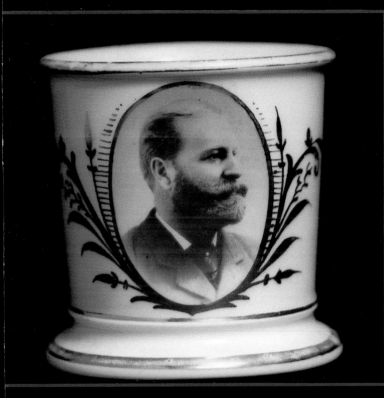

Non-personalized cameo. *Courtesy of Michael J. Griffin.*

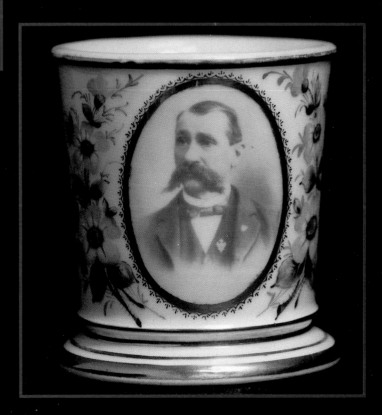

Non-personalized cameo, gent with K. of P. pin on lapel.
Courtesy of Michael J. Griffin.

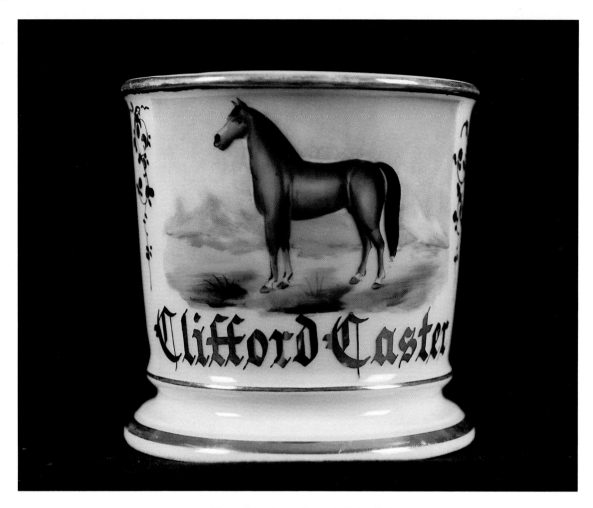

Horse. *Courtesy of Morris Pickerell, Jr.*

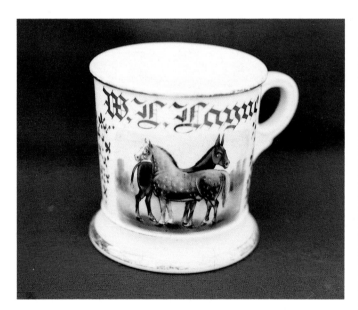

Horse and mule. *Courtesy of Bernard Lukco.*

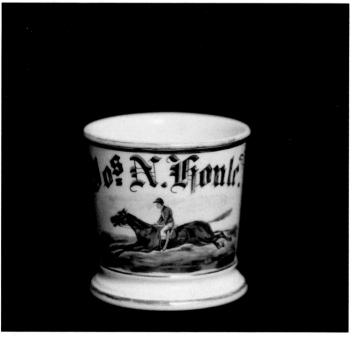

Jockey. *Courtesy of Roland F. Porter.*

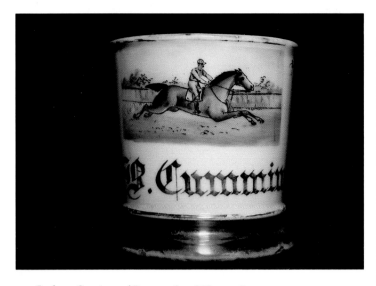

Jockey. *Courtesy of Raymond and Theresa Jones.*

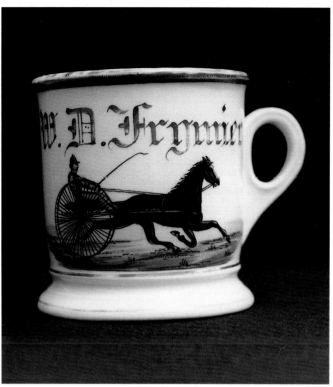

Trotter and driver. *Courtesy of Dr. Ralph Nix.*

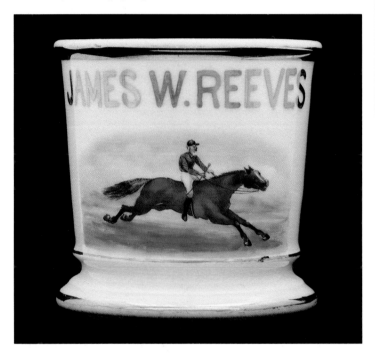

Jockey. *Anonymous.*

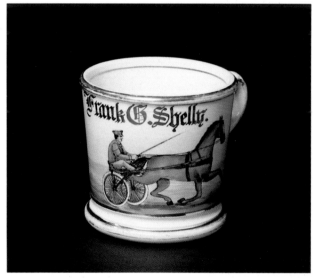

Trotter and driver. *Courtesy of Thomas and Penelope Nader.*

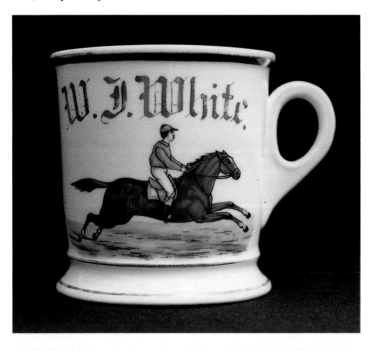

Jockey. *Courtesy of Dr. Ralph Nix.*

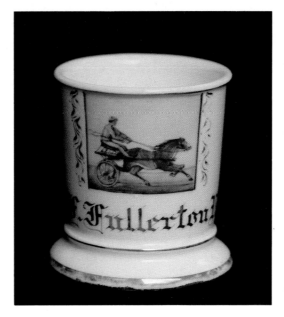
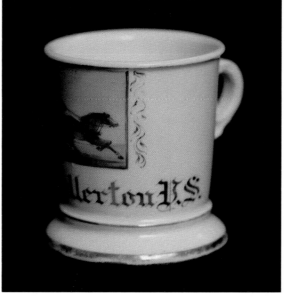

Trotter and driver, veterinary surgeon's mug. *Courtesy of Roland F. Porter.*

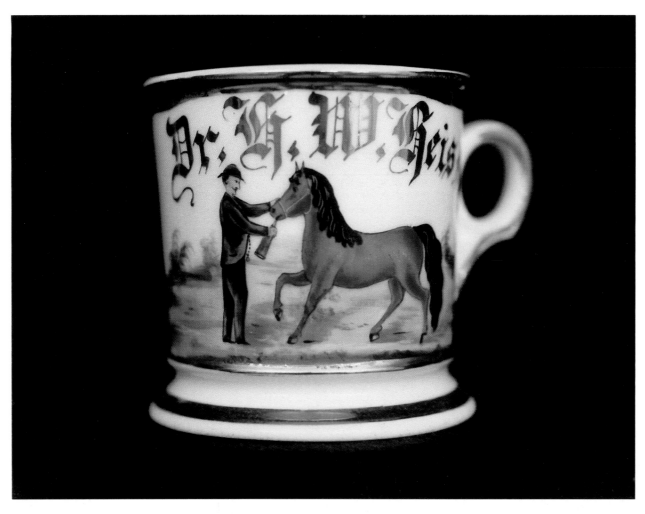

Doctor giving horse a tonic, veterinary. *Courtesy of Charles F. Kalb.*

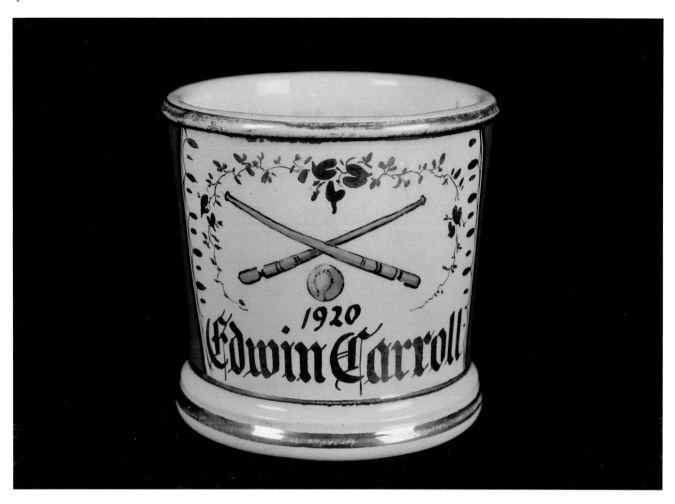

Baseball, bats and ball. *Courtesy of Morris Pickerell, Jr.*

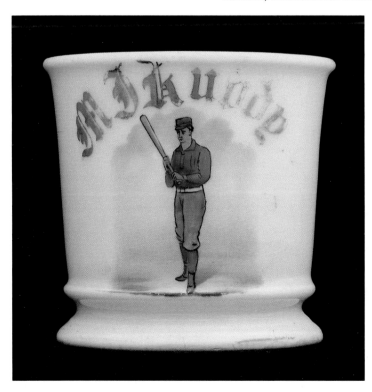

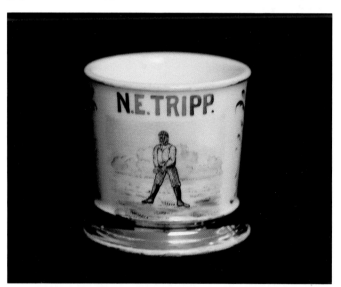

Baseball, catcher. *Courtesy of Roland F. Porter.*

Baseball, batter. *Courtesy of Anthony Gugliotti.*

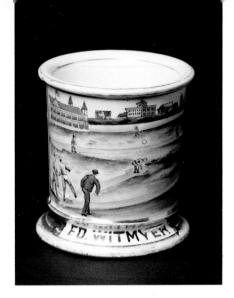

Baseball, umpire's mug with panorama. *Courtesy of Thomas and Penelope Nader.*

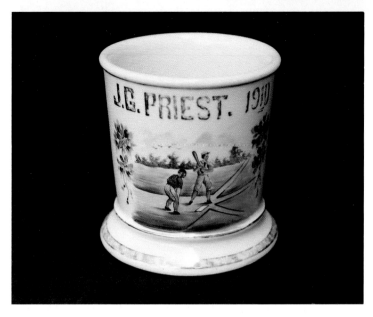

Baseball, professional, New York Yankee, rare. *Courtesy of Bernard Lukco.*

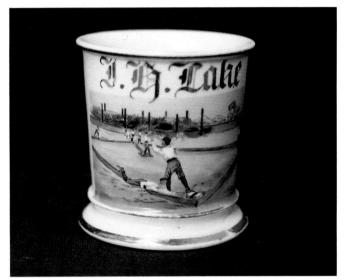

Baseball, full field. *Courtesy of Bernard Lukco.*

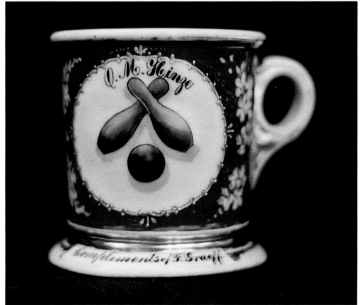

Bowling, ball and pins. *Courtesy of Dr. Ralph Nix.*

Bowling, bowling alley. *Courtesy of Charles F. Kalb.*

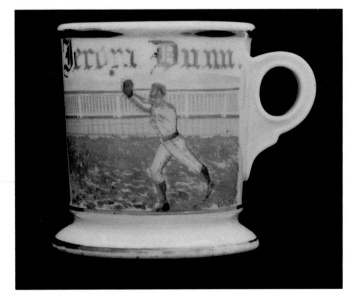

Baseball, outfielder. *Anonymous.*

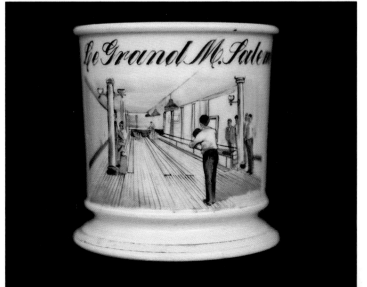

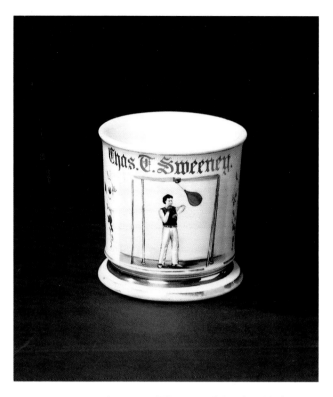

Boxer in training. *Courtesy of Thomas and Penelope Nader.*

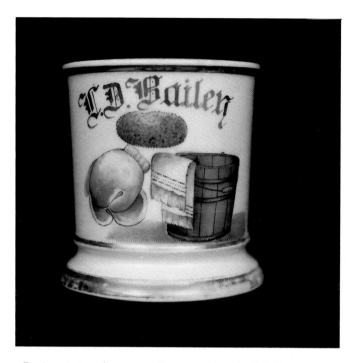

Boxing, trainer/manager. *Courtesy of Charles F. Kalb.*

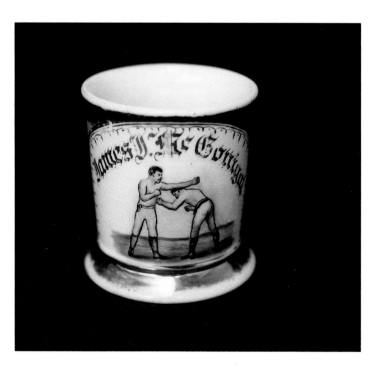

Boxer, bare knuckle fight. *Courtesy of Bernard Lukco.*

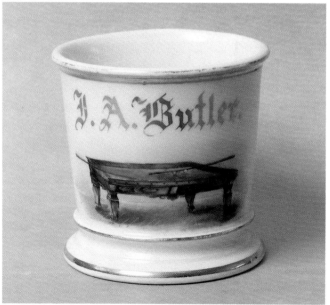

Pool table. *Courtesy of David Giese.*

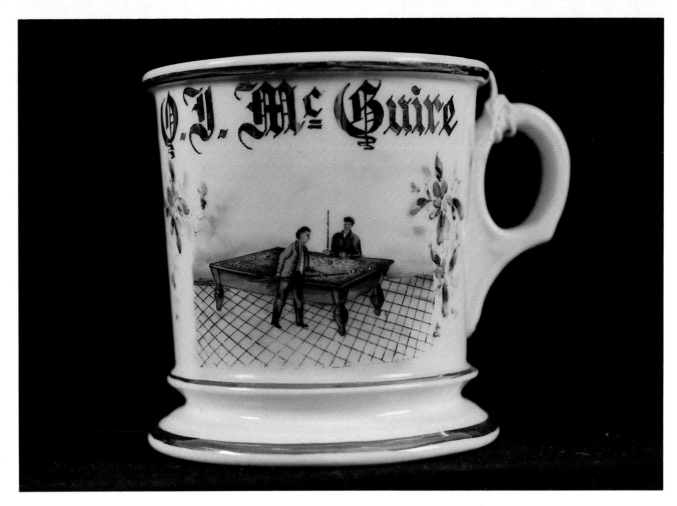

Pool players. *Courtesy of Morris Pickerell, Jr.*

Hunting and Fishing

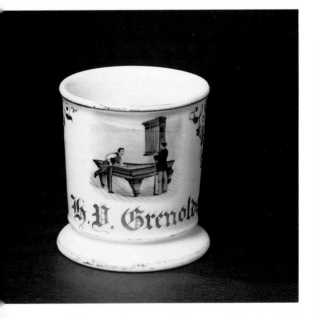

Pool players. *Courtesy of Thomas and Penelope Nader.*

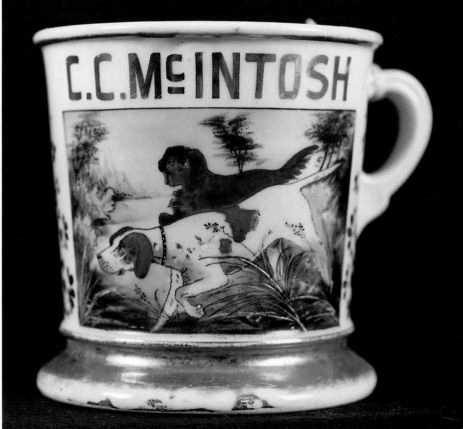

Hunting dogs. *Courtesy of Morris Pickerell, Jr.*

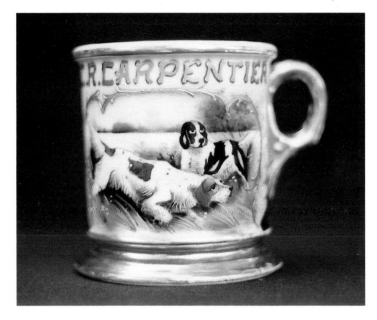

Hunting dogs. *Courtesy of Dr. Ralph Nix.*

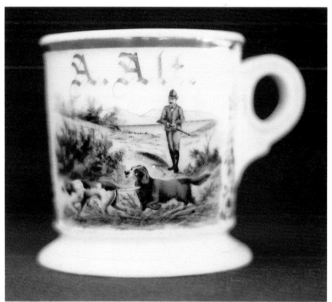

Hunter with dog. *Courtesy of Dr. Ralph Nix.*

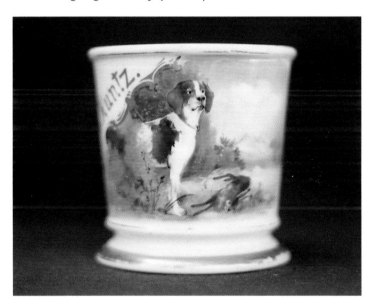

Hunting dog with rabbit. *Courtesy of Dr. Ralph Nix.*

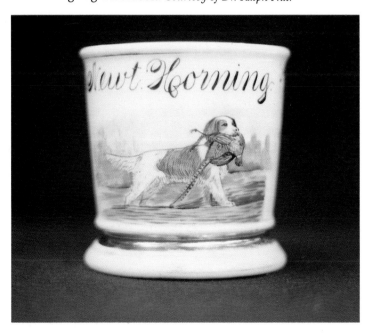

Hunter with dogs. *Courtesy of Dr. Ralph Nix.*

Hunting dog with pheasant. *Courtesy of Dr. Ralph Nix.*

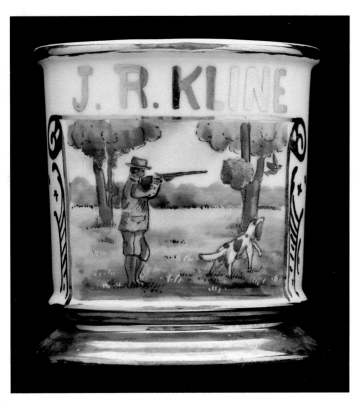

Hunter with dog on point. *Courtesy of Anthony Gugliotti.*

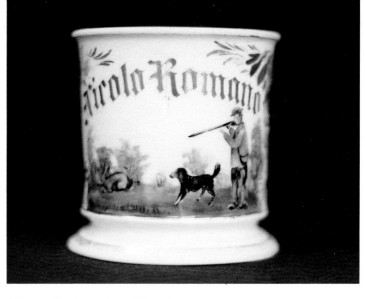

Hunter, dog on point, rabbit. *Courtesy of Dr. Ralph Nix.*

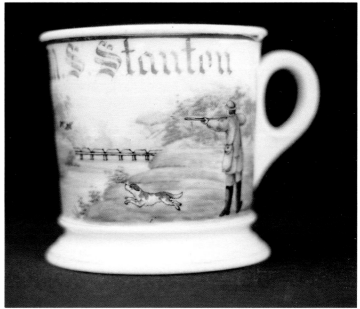

Hunter discharging gun. *Courtesy of Dr. Ralph Nix.*

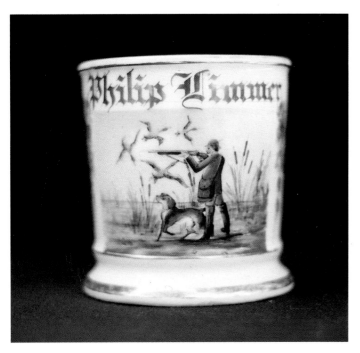

Bird hunter, dog on point. *Courtesy of Dr. Ralph Nix.*

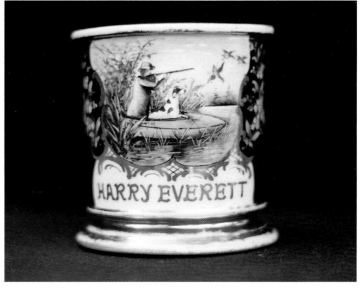

Hunter in skiff. *Courtesy of Dr. Ralph Nix.*

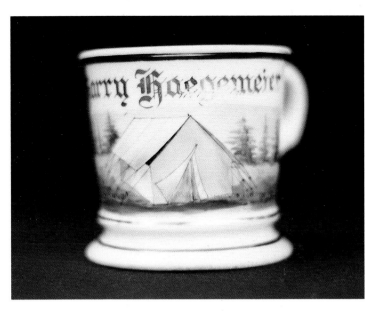

Hunt camp, tent. *Courtesy of Dr. Ralph Nix.*

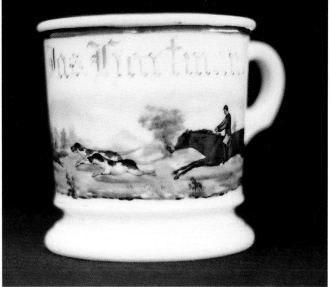

Mounted fox hunt.

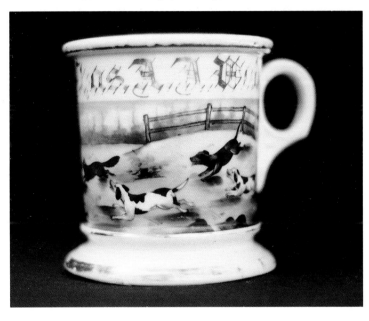

Fox hunt. *Courtesy of Dr. Ralph Nix.*

Fox hunt. *Courtesy of Dr. Ralph Nix.*

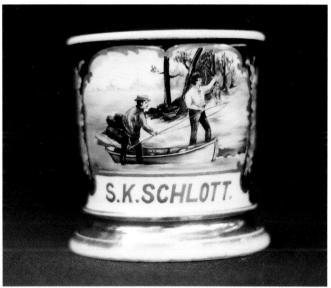

Sport fishing. *Courtesy of Dr. Ralph Nix.*

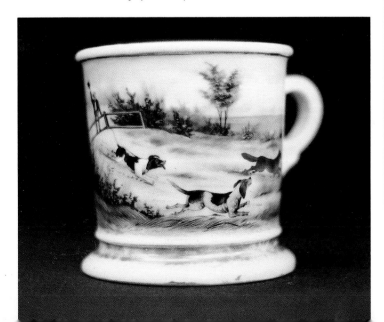

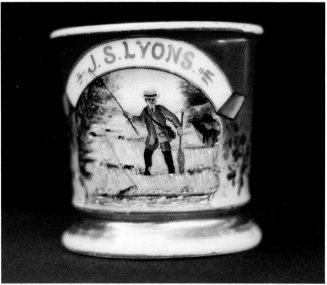

White water sport fishing. *Courtesy of Dr. Ralph Nix.*

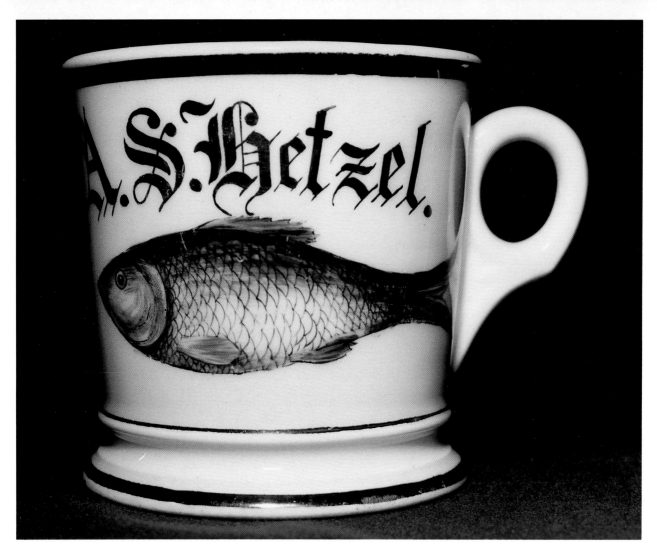

Fish, Shad. *Courtesy of Raymond and Theresa Jones.*

Soldiers and Shooters

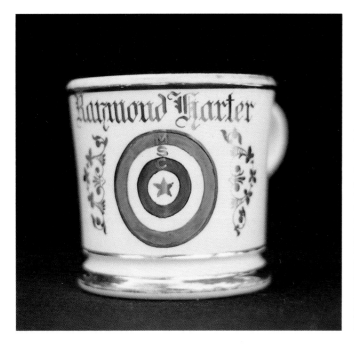

Target. *Courtesy of Dr. Ralph Nix.*

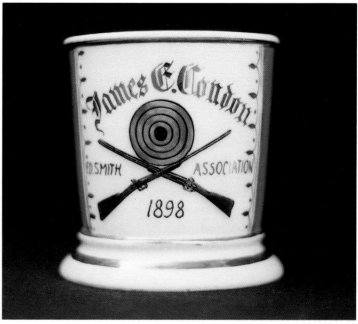

Target club. *Courtesy of Dr. Ralph Nix.*

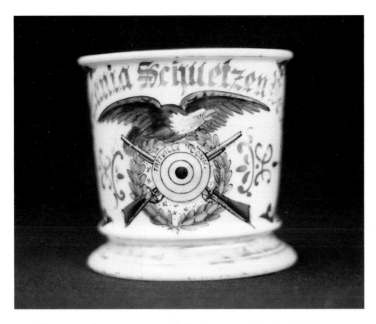

German-American target club. *Courtesy of Dr. Ralph Nix.*

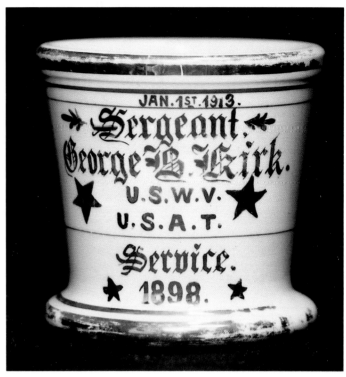

Sergeant, Spanish-American War veteran. *Courtesy of Michael J. Griffin.*

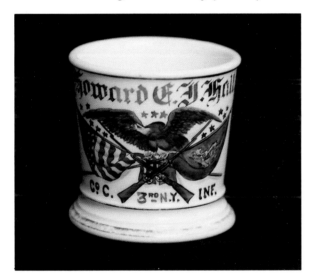

3rd N.Y. Infantry, Co. *Courtesy of Roland F. Porter.*

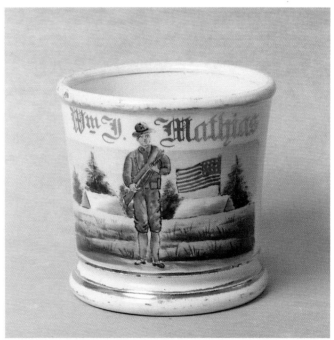

Soldier, 1900s era. *Courtesy of David Giese.*

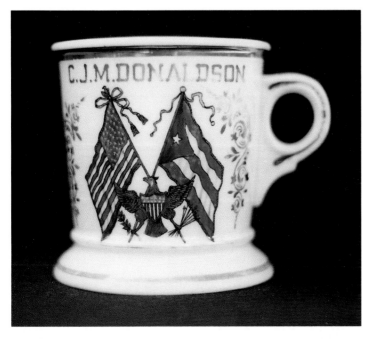

Spanish-American War vet. *Courtesy of Dr. Ralph Nix.*

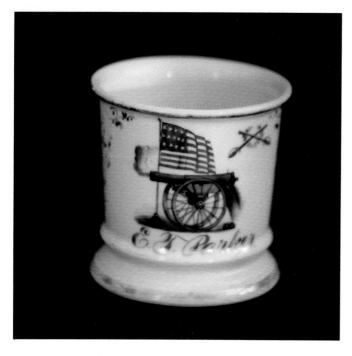

Flag, cannon and crossed swords. *Courtesy of Bernard Lukco.*

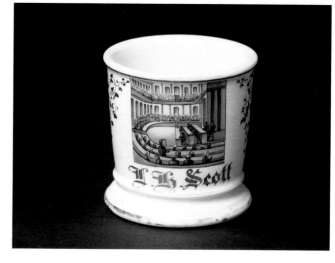

Senate, senator or politician's mug. *Courtesy of Thomas and Penelope Nader.*

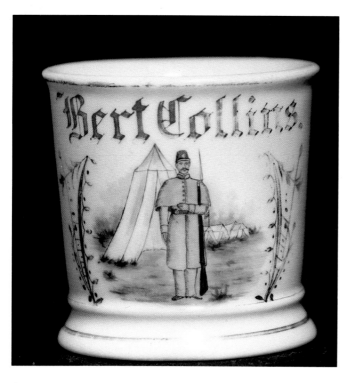

Civil War soldier. *Courtesy of Michael J. Griffin.*

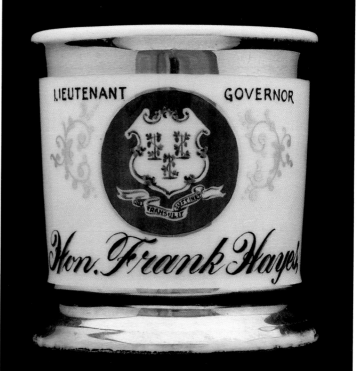

Lt. Governor, state of Connecticut seal. *Courtesy of Anthony Gugliotti.*

Biplane, pilot, 1922. *Courtesy of Bernard Lukco.*

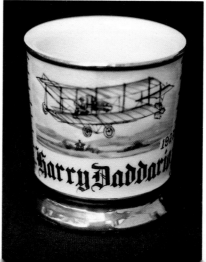

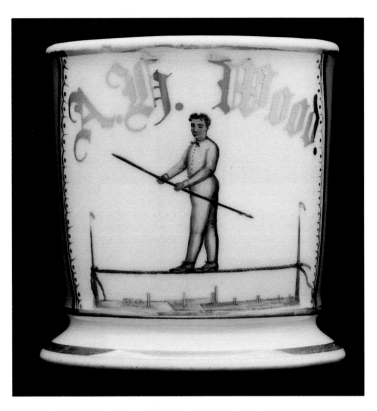

Tightrope walker. *Courtesy of Anthony Gugliotti.*

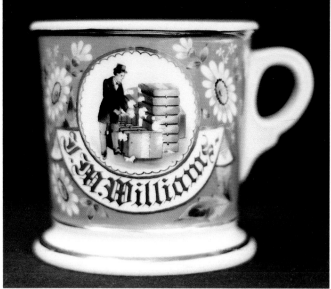

Cotton merchant, inspecting bales. *Courtesy of Dr. Ralph Nix.*

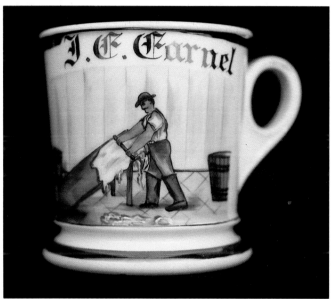

Hide tanner, working. *Courtesy of Charles F. Kalb.*

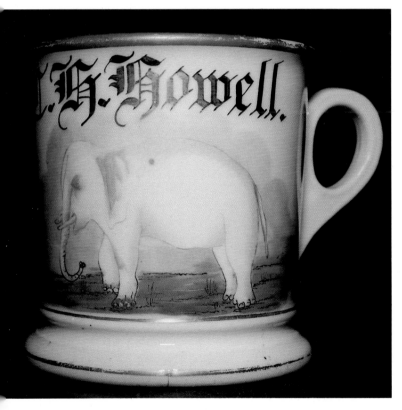

Elephant, circus related. *Courtesy of Raymond and Theresa Jones.*

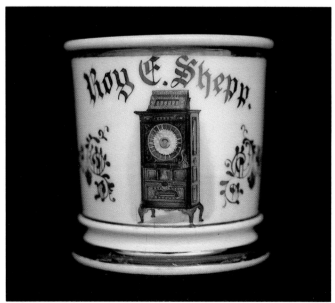

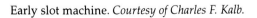

Early slot machine. *Courtesy of Charles F. Kalb.*

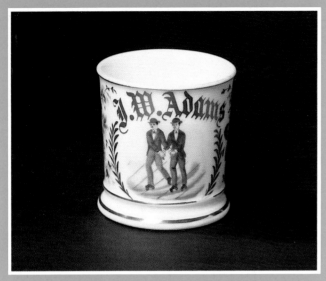

Roller skaters, two men holding hands. *Courtesy of Thomas and Penelope Nader.*

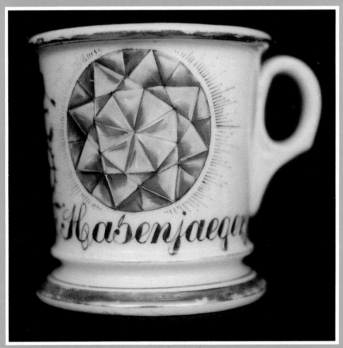

Diamond cutter. *Courtesy of Charles F. Kalb.*

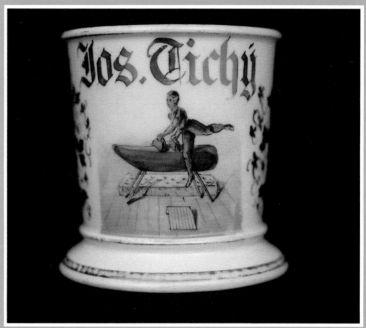

Gymnast at horse. *Courtesy of Charles F. Kalb.*

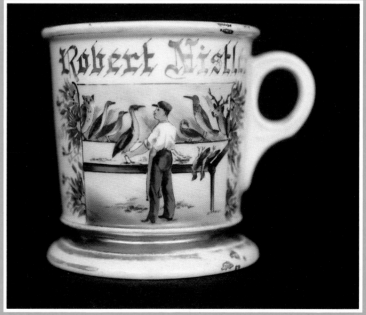

Taxidermist. *Courtesy of Charles F. Kalb.*

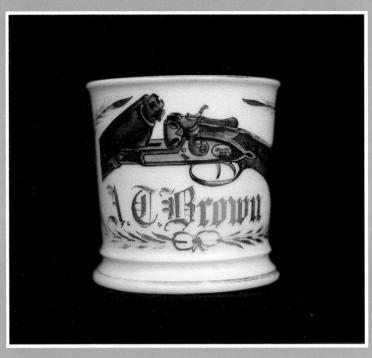

Gunsmith. *Courtesy of Charles F. Kalb.*

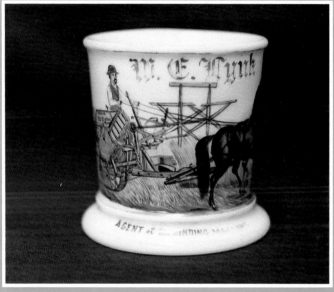

Binding machine agent, Deering Co. *Courtesy of Bernard Lukco.*

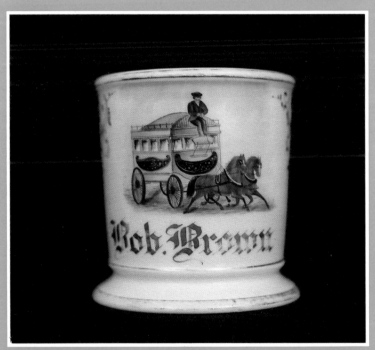

Horse drawn omnibus. *Courtesy of Charles F. Kalb.*

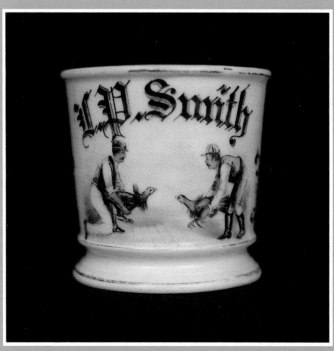

Cock fighter's mug. *Courtesy of Charles F. Kalb.*

Specialized Collections

Certain collectors are attracted to one special subject or particular type of mug. I have two examples here of specialized collections.

Nautical Mug Collection

Ray and Theresa Jones are advanced Occupational collectors, but their main collecting interests lies in mugs with Nautical themes. Ray was a Naval aviator during World War II. Since then he has had an interest in ocean-related collectibles.

Shown here, is the finest boat and ship mug collection known. As with most first generation collectors, it has taken over 30 years to acquire this collection.

Jone's Nautical Collection

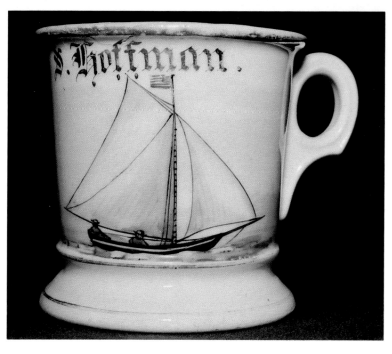

Sail yacht.

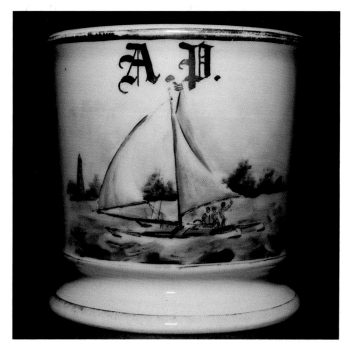

Catamaran.

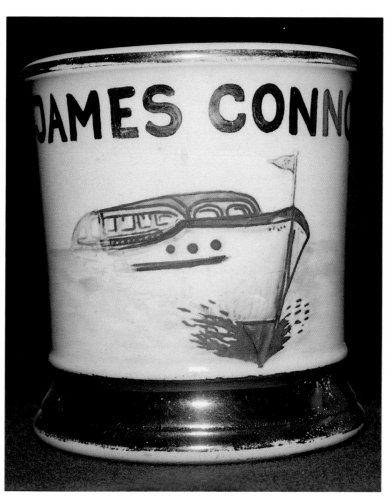

Motor boat.

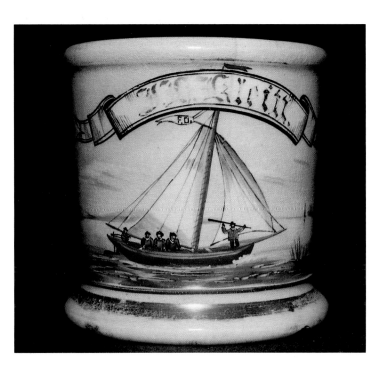

Early whaling boat.

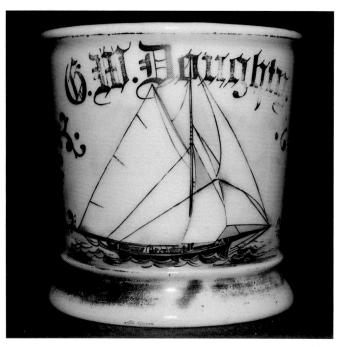

Hudson River sloop.

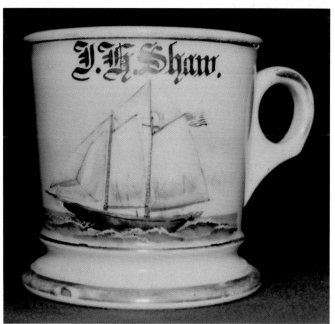

Two-masted schooner.

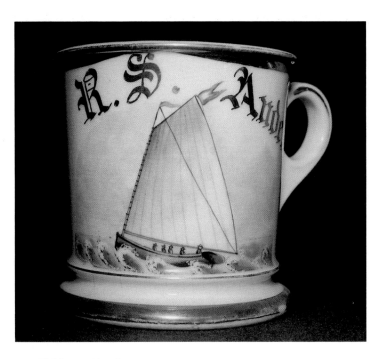

Fishing cat boat.

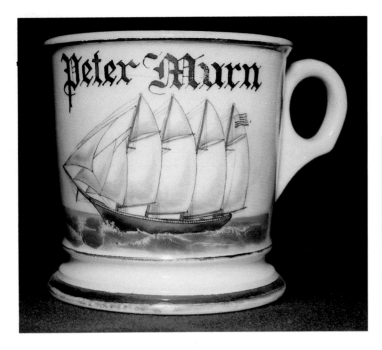

Four-masted schooner.

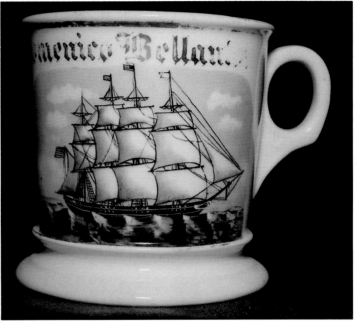

Four-masted ship.

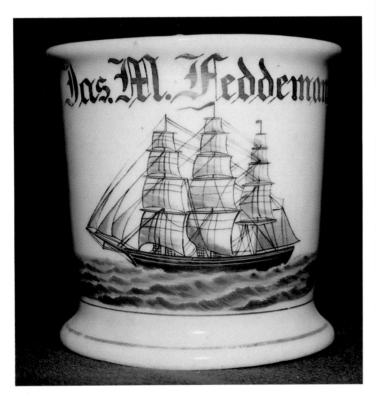

Three-masted ship.

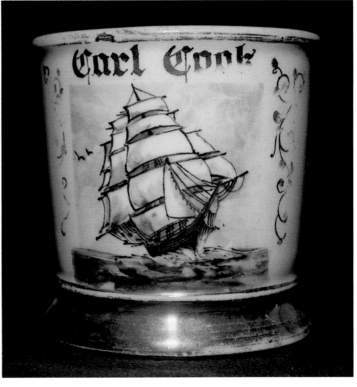

Four-masted ship.

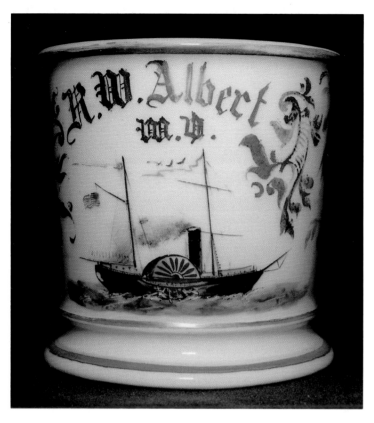

Paddle wheel steam ship.

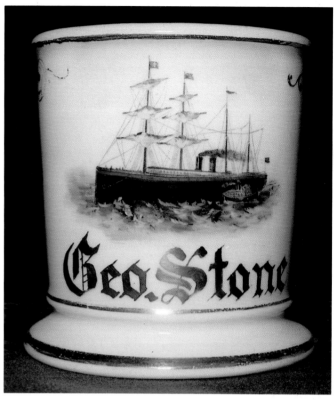

Steam/sail passenger liner.

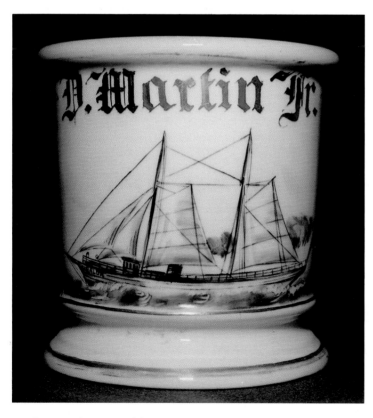

Screw-type steam ship.

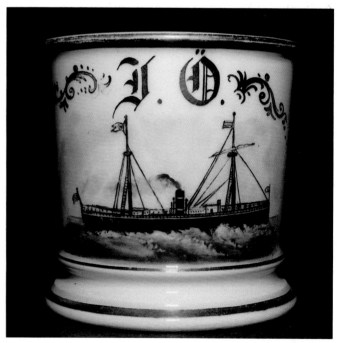

Early steam cargo ship with sail.

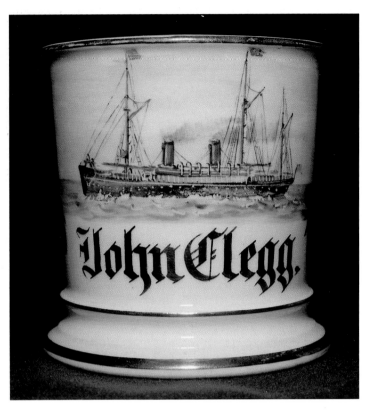

Early cargo passenger ship.

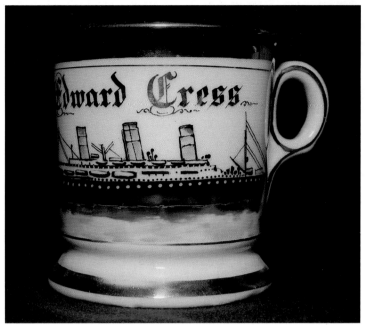

Ocean liner.

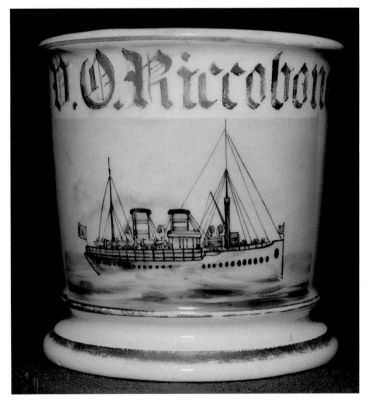

Large cargo passenger ship.

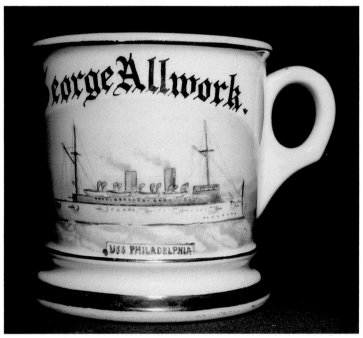

1890s cruiser, U.S.S. Philadelphia.

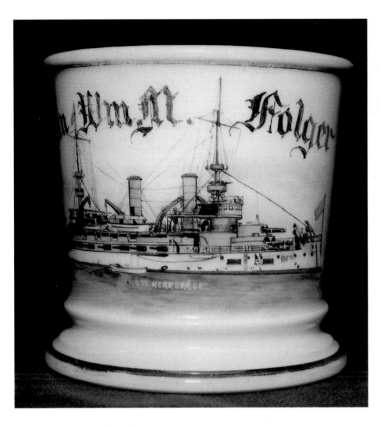

1890s battleship, Kearsage.

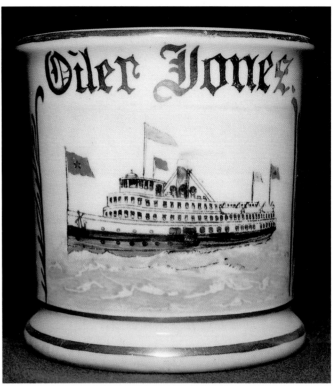

Great Lakes passenger/cargo ship.

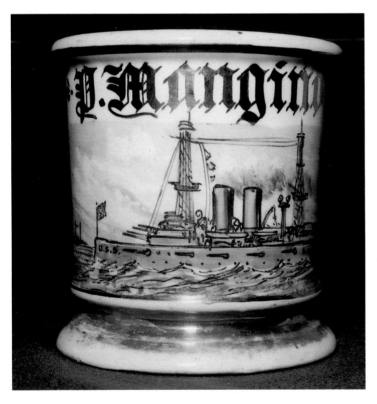

1910 battleship.

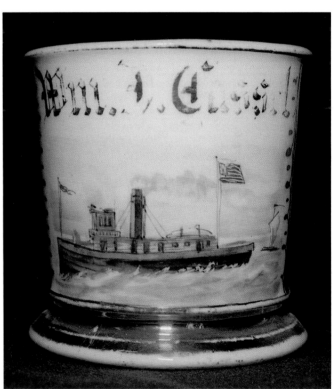

Early tug, wooden hull.

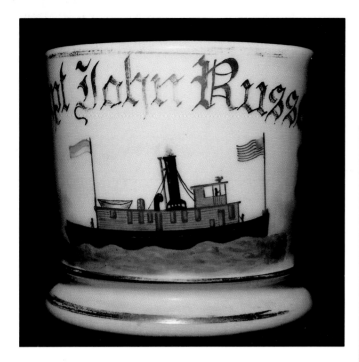

Later tug, steel hull.

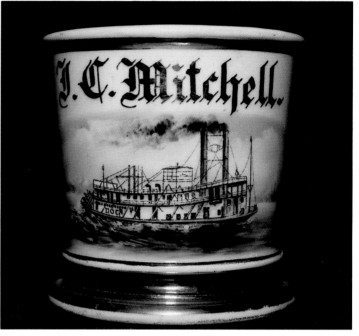

Steam paddle wheel, large river steamer.

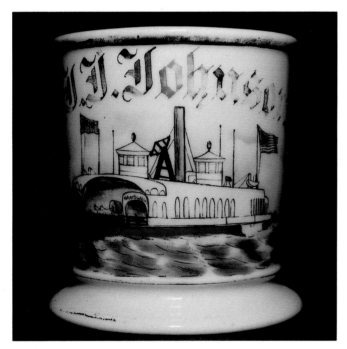

Large bay or river ferry.

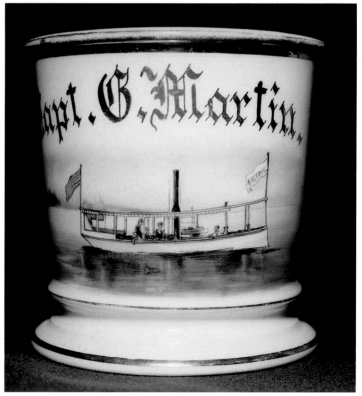

Lake passenger launch.

166

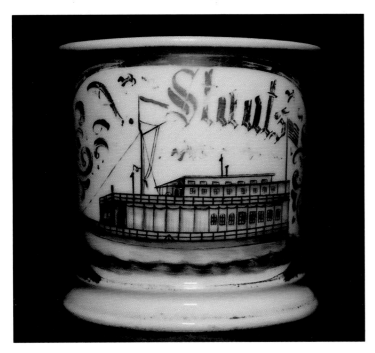

Early work or prison barge.

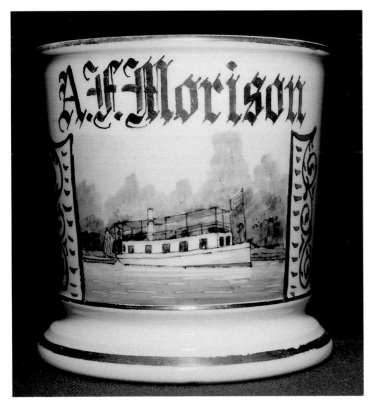

Lake passenger launch.

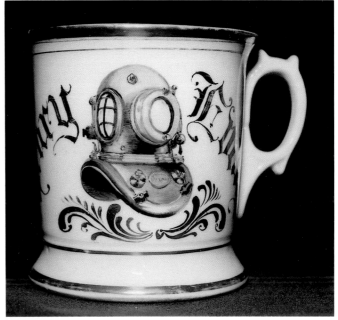

World War I diver's helmet.

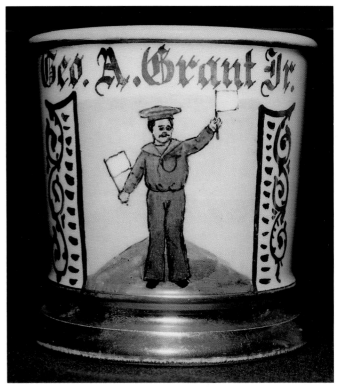

1890s sailor, sending semaphore code.

Character Mugs

Character mugs were imported from England and Germany from 1900 to 1925. They were sold through large department stores, not through barber suppliers.

Some mugs have the shape of a subject's head, others have raised figures on a blank, and some are made along the same lines as Scuttle Mugs.

Many of these mugs were manufactured as "go-withs". This means that several different china items, such as pitchers and tobacco jars, all have the same subject. Slight variations and sizes would determine the particular use. The most sought after mugs are those with the matching shaving brush. Another popular mug is an Englishman with an ape on the opposite end. The mug could be used either way. Two manufacturers of these particular mugs were Schaffer and Vater and E. Bone. Both of these were German.

The foremost collector of character mugs is Dave Giese. He has spent the last 25 years putting together the finest collection known. Examples from that collection are shown here.

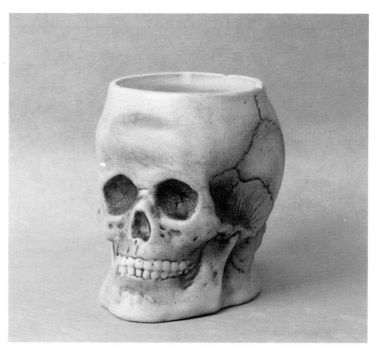

Skull.

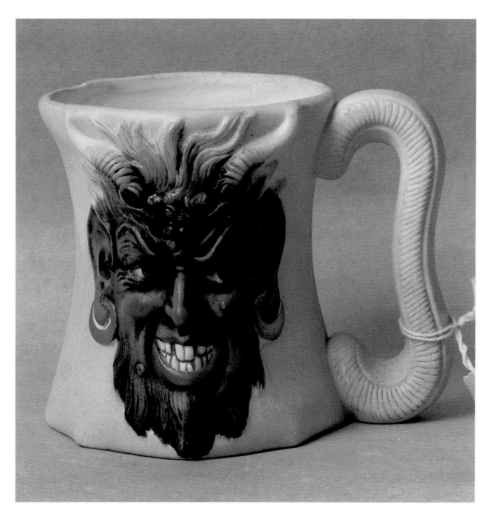

Raised design, devil.

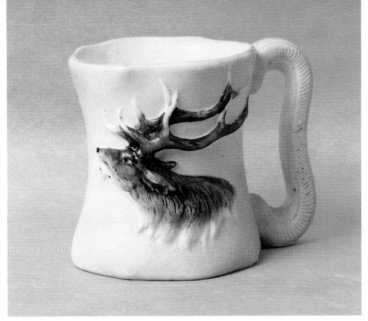

Raised design, elk.

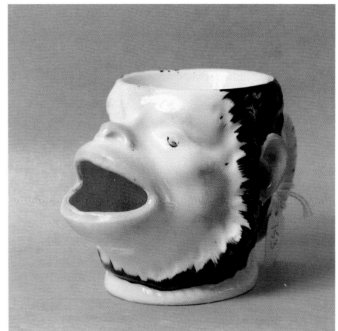

Monkey.

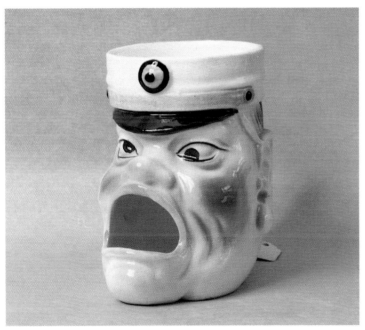

Foreign legionnaire.

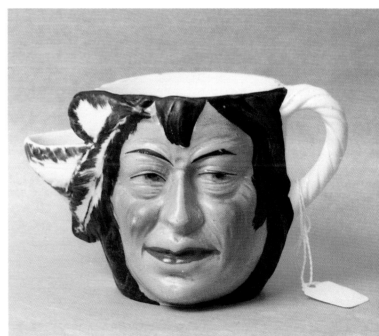

Indian.

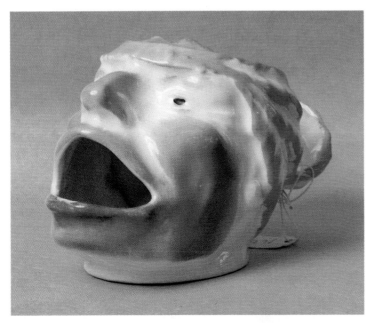

English man.

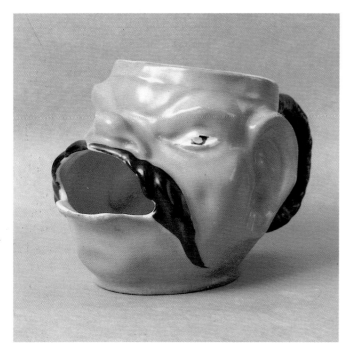

Chinese man.

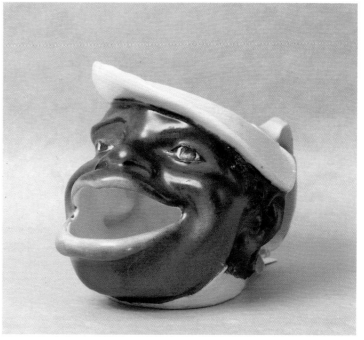

Afro-American with cap.

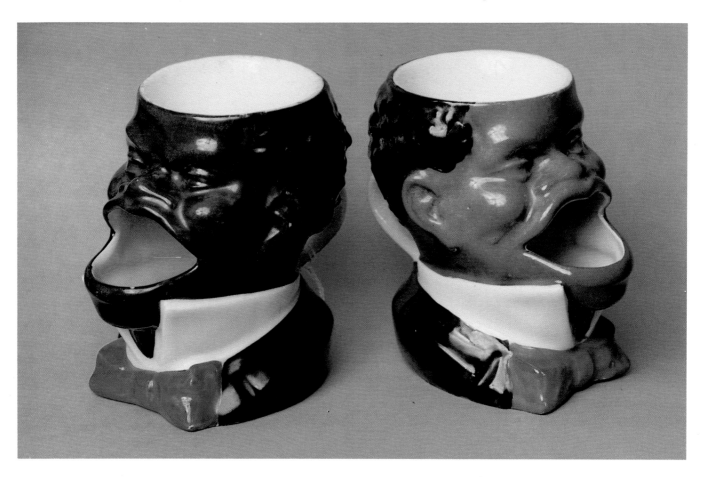

Afro-American, dark and light skin examples.

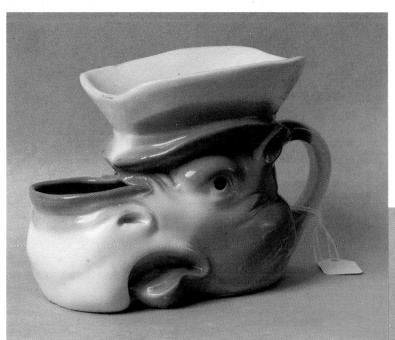

Rhino.

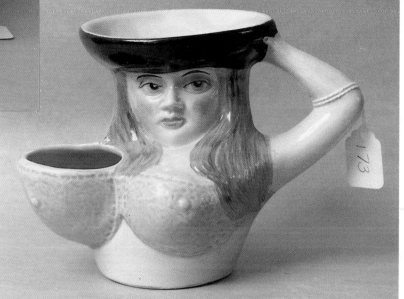

"Judy" mug.

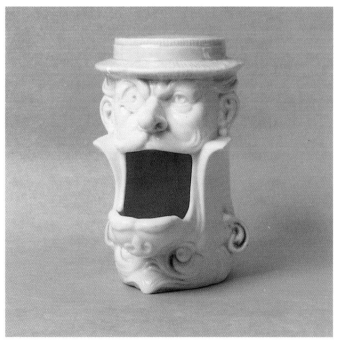

English man and reverse ape.

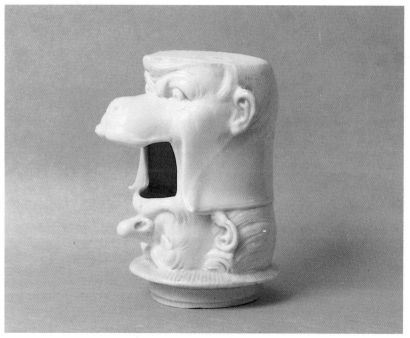

Ape and reverse Englishman.

171

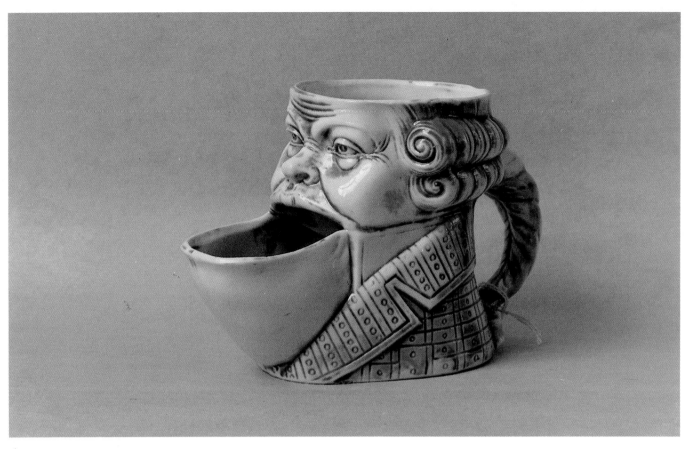

Englishman with wig.

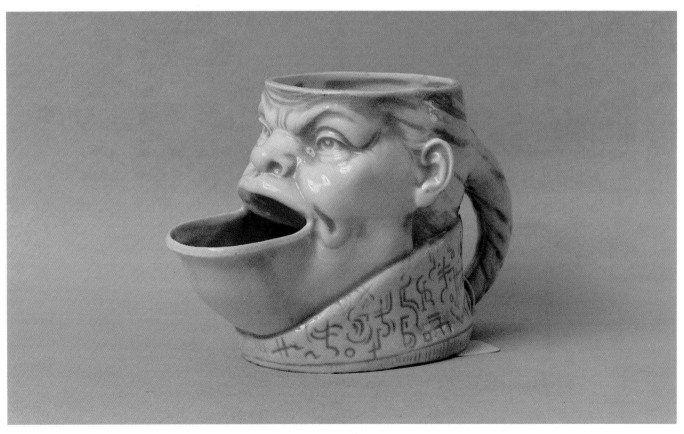

Chinese man.

172

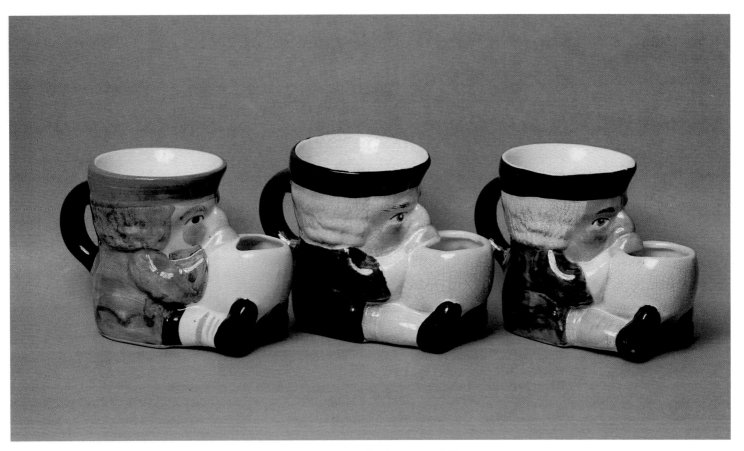

Toby mugs, yellow, green and blue.

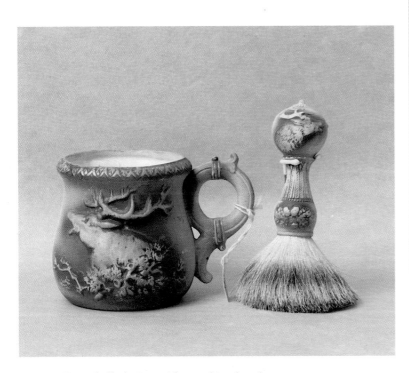

Raised elk design with matching brush.

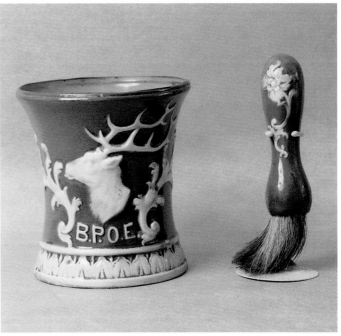

B.P.O.E., raised design with brush.

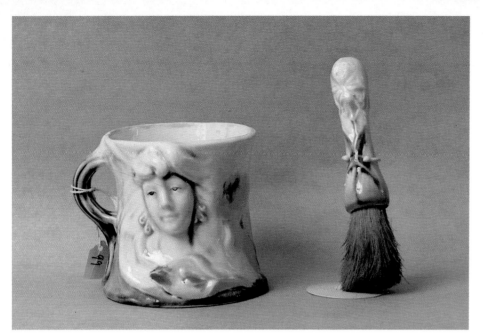

Majolica, girl with flowing hair with brush.

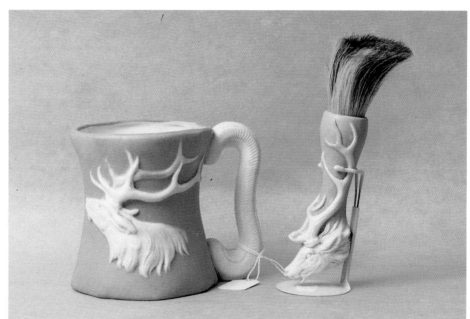

Raised design elk with matching brush.

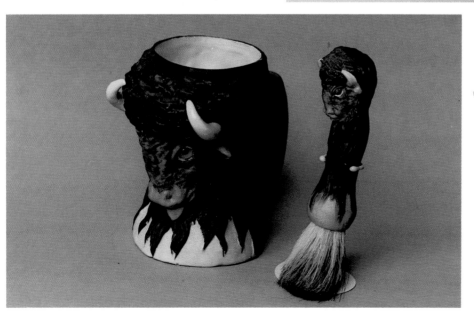

Buffalo head with matching brush.

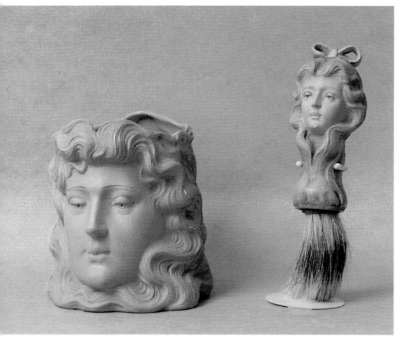

Blond girl with flowing hair, with matching brush.

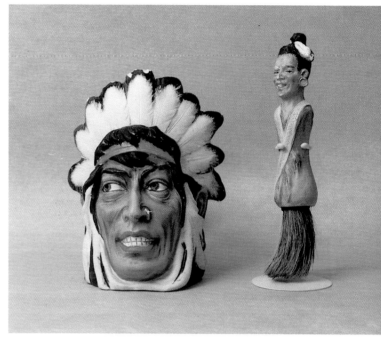

Indian "chief" with "princess" brush.

Devil with matching brush.

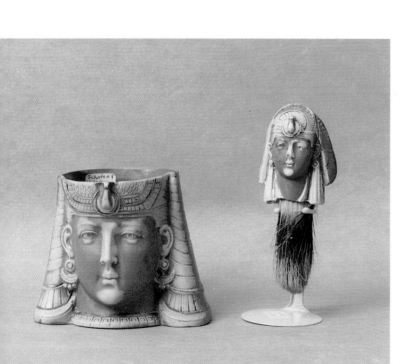

Egyptian with matching brush.

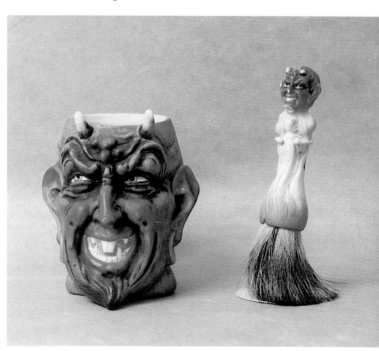

Artistic Interpretation

Here are three mugs that represent the same pastime, deer hunting. The second and third mugs have unusual and desired graphics. The artists have given us scenes that make us appreciate their skill and labor.

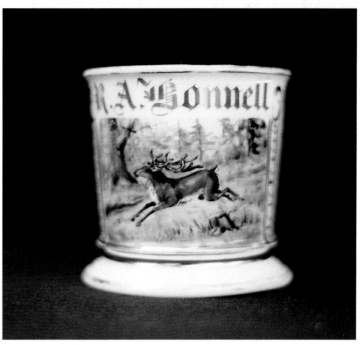

Here is a standard illustration of a buck running through the woods. It is considered an Occupational, but there is nothing special about this. There are similar decal scenes on non-personalized mugs.

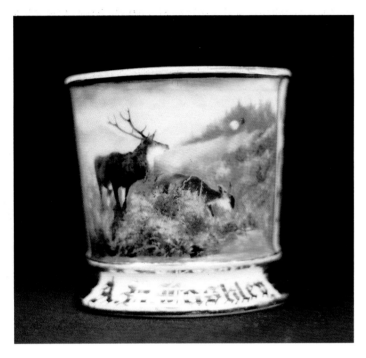

A buck and doe have come to a pool for a drink. The buck has sensed danger and has his head raised and his ears extended. Unknown to the deer, a hunter has been waiting in the distant tree line. He has aimed and shot, a white puff of smoke from his gun can be seen. What happens next is up to us. Some would assume that the buck will fall, but the hunter is far away and the buck is already alert. If the shot is a miss, both deer will bolt from the scene and escape to safety.

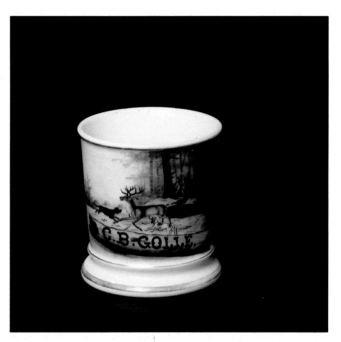

This mug shows the end of the hunt. The deer has been chased by the dogs and has been run to ground. His tongue protrudes from his mouth in exhaustion. The dogs have him at bay, but aren't attacking, as he could still inflict serious wounds with his antlers. The hunter, who has been following the dogs, is now emerging from the woods. Within a minute or so the hunt will be over. The artist gives us realistic and absolute scene. We know the hunter will be successful.

Details

Here is a mug that needs a close look, perhaps with a magnifying glass. At first glance it appears to be the watch of a railroad employee. He would use the watch as a symbol of punctuality. But under a lens, it reveals a "Rockford Railroad watch". This is the mug of a Rockford Railroad pocketwatch salesman, probably a "one of a kind".

Always take a second or third look at a mug, convince yourself what the details mean. Now you can make an educated purchase.

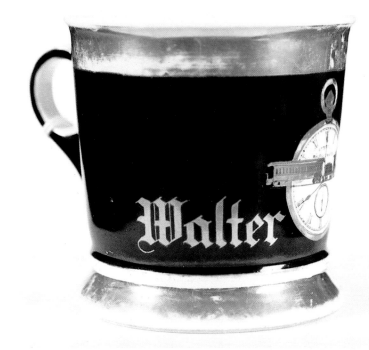

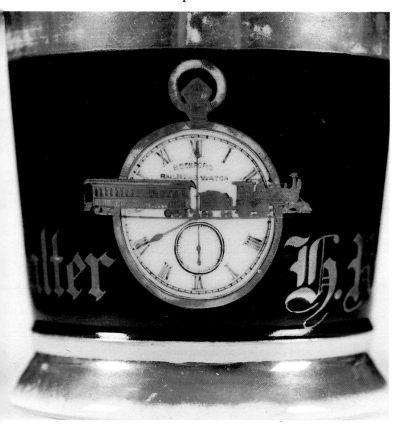

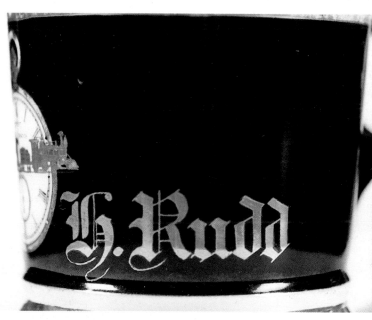

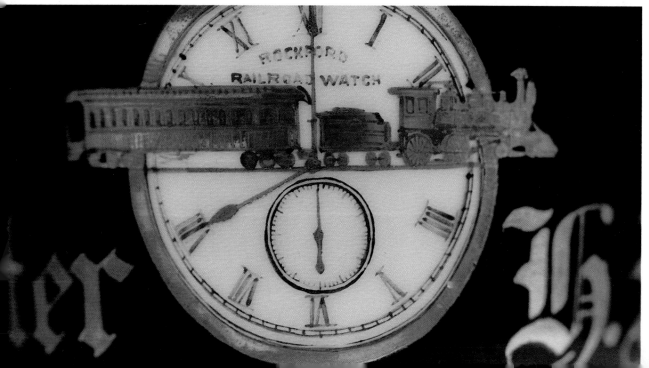

Chapter 4
Non-Personalized
and Reproduction Shaving Mugs

This section will deal with all non-personalized mugs and reproductions.

The Sears Roebuck catalog was the shopping mall of the 1890s. Anything you could possibly want and sitting on a table in your parlor. And shaving mugs were among the thousands of items that they sold. These were not the $2 or $3 mugs you bought from the barber. They cost about 25 cents or 50 cents and were generally smaller. They had another feature which made them different, a soap drain within the mug. These drains could hold half a bar of shaving soap or a brush, whatever the owner desired.

In rural America no barber shop was available and a trip to town was a once-a-week venture, probably to attend church on Sunday. So a man had a bath and a shave on Saturday night. He would shave himself if he had a steady hand; if not, his wife probably had the chore. These mugs were usually touched up with decals, not totally hand painted illustrations.

General stores also sold these mugs. They are numerous and can be found at swap meets and tag sales today. They are not to be confused with moustache cups, which also have an insert.

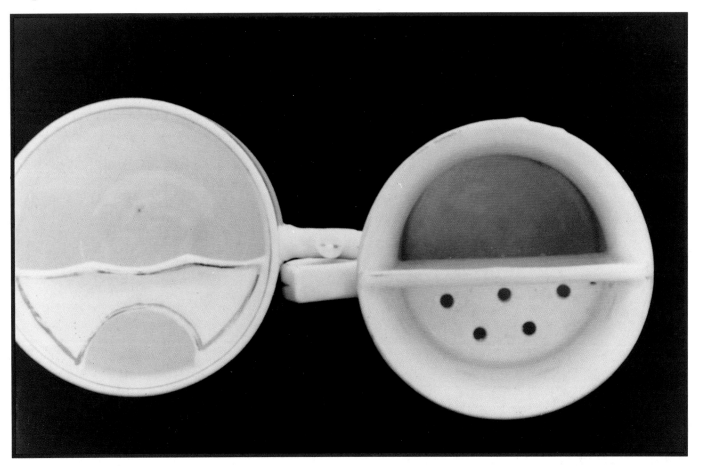

On the left is the moustache cup and on the right is the shaving mug. The holes allow excess water to drain into the mug.

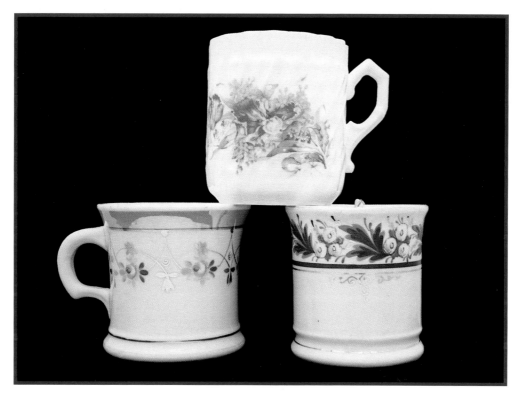

Some non-personalized shaving mugs.

Trigger Blanks

Another type of mug is the "trigger blank." It gets its name from its handle, which resembles the trigger guard on certain guns. Trigger blanks usually were decorated with a better grade of decal than soap drain mugs. The china is of a better grade also. I have seen a few Occupationals on trigger blanks but they don't have the professional quality of the barber shop blank. They are probably attempts by some local person to get into the mug decorating business.

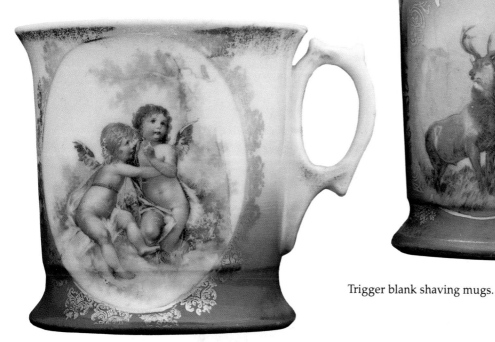

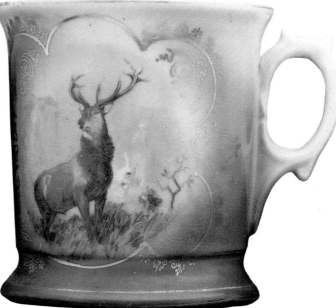

Trigger blank shaving mugs.

179

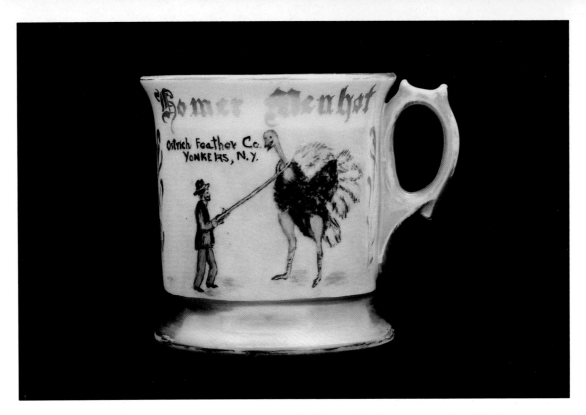

An Occupational mug on a trigger blank.

Scuttle Mugs

This is another mail order decal mug, and quite functional. It has a large drain and a slot to hold the brush. These mugs are sought by certain collectors and the price can rise into the $100 range. There are several modern reproductions of these mugs. One is a hand holding cards, another has a view of the statue of liberty. The examples shown here are authentic.

Three examples of scuttle mugs.

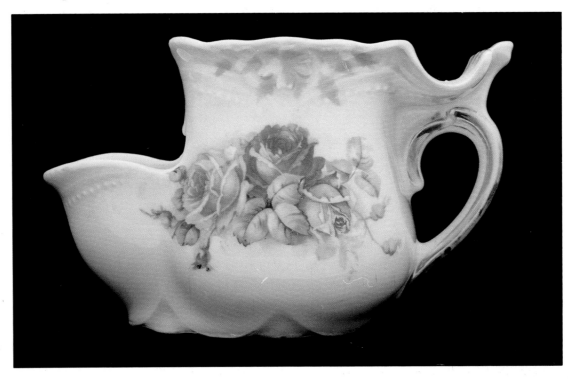

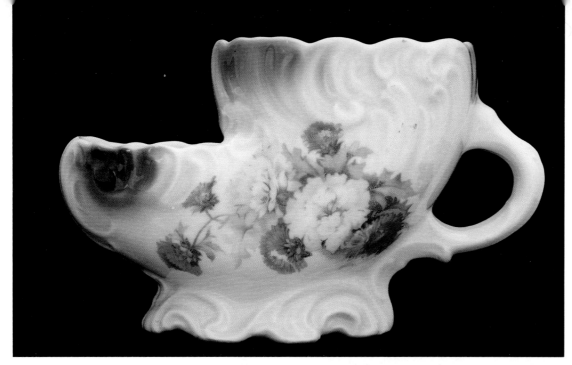

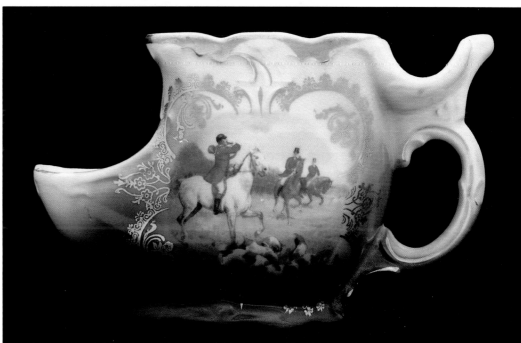

Fine China Mugs

Several foreign and one American china company (Lennox), made a fine, thin china shaving mug. These resemble the dishes and tea cups that were the standard china place settings of the day. These thin mugs were designed to be used at home, as they couldn't take the beatings of daily barber shop use.

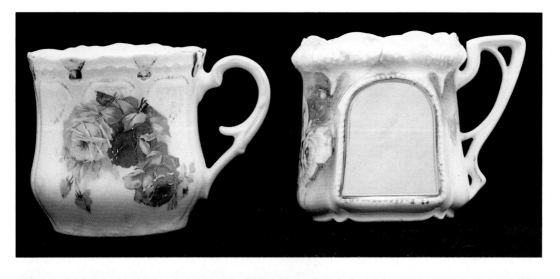

Two examples of fine china shaving mugs. A small mirror was added to the mug on the right.

Raised China

These mugs had decorations of flowers raised from the china itself, then painted and sometimes gilded. They are usually soap drain mugs.

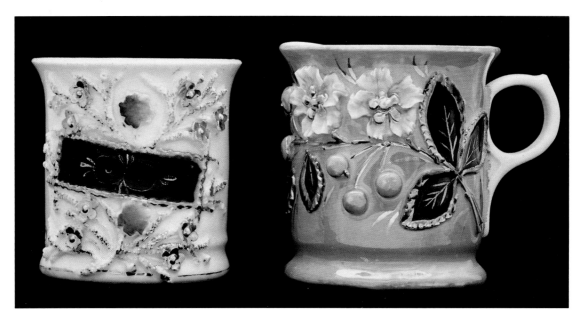

Raised china mugs.

Silver Plated Mugs

Some of these mugs were sold through the supplier's catalogs. Some are dated and personalized. They are numerous and many collectors pass on them because they aren't considered folk art.

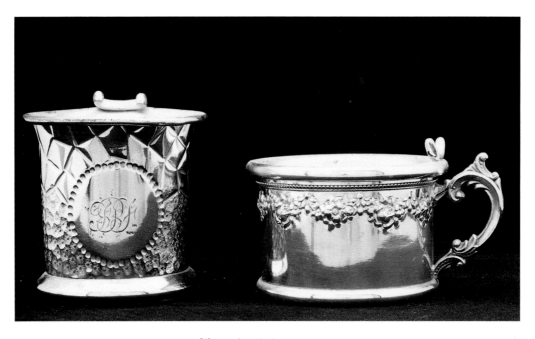

Silver plated shaving mugs.

After Era Mugs

In the 1940s a barber shop customer would become intrigued with an old rack of mugs, that was on display in the shop. They would inquire as to where they could have their own mug made. The barber may have known of a distributor who could still have a mug produced. Since the era of the mug died in the 1920s, this may have been difficult.

The customer may have never used his mug, but just wanted to see his name among the others on the rack.

The two mugs shown here are on the same style blank, the letters "JHK" appear on the bottom. The artistry of the Floral is not up to the quality of the early mugs and the blank is a heavy eggshell white similar to the "Sportsman" mugs. The mayor mug is dated, so we know when this was made. These mugs aren't reproductions, they are simply the best that could be produced at this late period. Both of these mugs came from the Waterbury, Connecticut area.

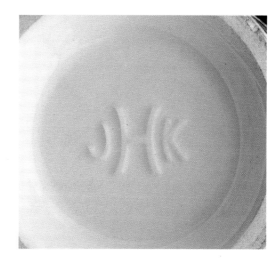

Both of the after era mugs shown are marked JHK on the bottom.

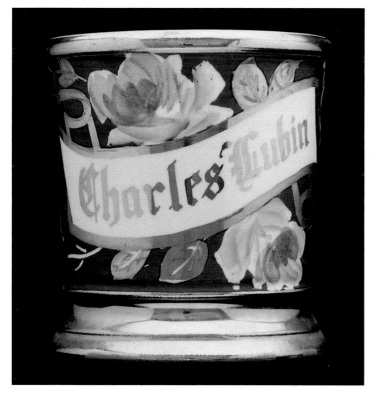

A Floral mug of a late date.

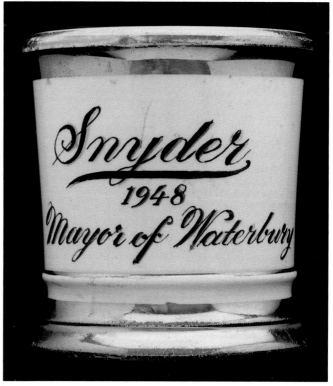

A mug for the mayor of Waterbury, dated 1948.

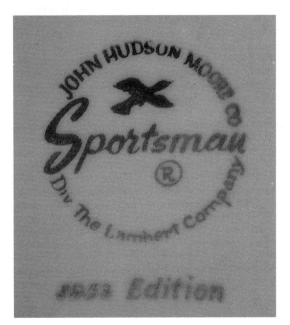

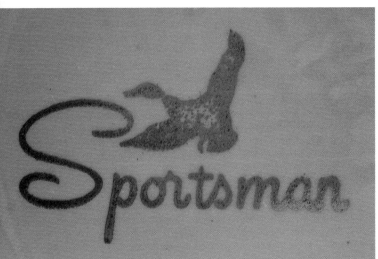

Sportsman Mugs

In the early 1950s many people found an interest in collecting shaving mugs. At this same time the Lambert company (now Warner-Lambert) had hand-painted mugs produced to be sold with their shaving soap in the retail market.

Many different varieties exist, but they all have two common characteristics. They have the word "the" before each occupation and the illustrations have a "watercolor" look to them, not as bright as original mugs.

The early issues are the most desired. These are stamped on the bottom by a duck in flight and the word "Sportsman," or a small circle with the duck and logo and a stamp stating "1953 Edition". Sportsman mugs were produced for about two years.

Sportsman mugs are becoming more difficult to find as they represent a pleasing and a much cheaper form of collecting. Being forty years old they are somewhat of an antique. Sometimes Sportsman mugs are sold for over $100, but a more realistic price is $50-$75.

The Sportsman mugs included "The": Autoist, Broker, Sea Captain, Doctor, Engineer, Fireman, Farmer, Horseman, Ice man, Lawyer, Policeman, Salesman, Father, Rancher, Bartender, Musician, Pharmacist, Dentist, Oilman, Butcher, Barber, and Barbershop quartet. The "Father" and the "Horseman" are the most common. The "Bartender" is difficult to find.

The stamps of early issue Sportsman mugs.

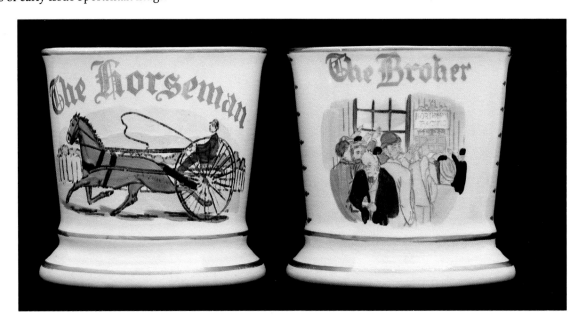

"The Horseman" and "The Broker" Sportsman mugs.

184

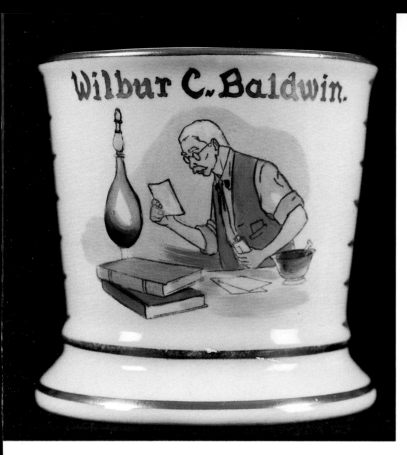

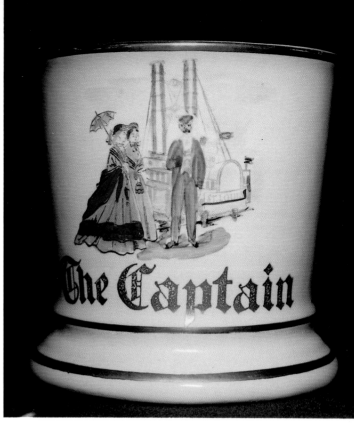

Sportsman mugs could be ordered from the factory personalized. These are seldom seen, but they present the problem of passing as a real Occupational. Here is an example of a pharmacist. Mugs personalized with "John A. Brown" are display examples.

Sometimes the graphics of a Sportsman can differ from the standard variety. Here is the "Captain" mug, with the unusual feature of the two women in the illustration. These mugs may have been experimental types, with only a few examples being produced.

Mugged by a Mug

Looks beautiful, doesn't it? Would you like to buy it for $600 or $700? If you have, you had better go to your medicine cabinet and get some Maalox, you're going to need it.

Yes, it's a reproduction, and a very good one. These mugs were manufactured in the early 1950s. One story is that they could be ordered from a mortuary distributor.

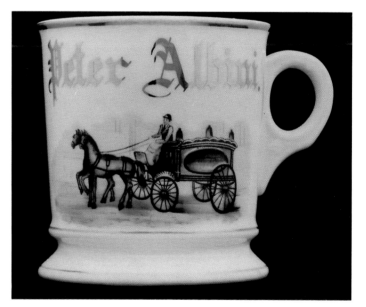

The letters "KF" appear on the base in red. The illustration shown here is the only known type. And the mug usually is found with no name. This particular mug had a name fired on it to make it look real.

I have seen an example of this for sale. And it was correctly identified as a reproduction. The price was $100.

I have also seen an example, on which someone tried to remove the "KF" off of the bottom. This was an attempt to fool a new collector, all advanced collectors know of this mug. And now so do you.

The KF on the bottom of the hearse mug.

Silk Screen

This Japanese import shows various trades and occupations. Sometimes they are confused with "Sportsman" mugs, but that these don't use the word "the" before the occupation. They are illustrated with a silk screen process and they have no hand decoration. They are very common.

These mugs are more trouble to dealers than collectors. A dealer should never sell reproductions with the exception of the "Sportsman" series. It tends to hurt their reputation, and are not worth the trouble of going from show to show trying to sell them.

I got a call from someone wanting to sell their "school teacher" Occupational. When I asked what the name on the mug was, and they said "teacher" I had to tell them the sad truth, they own a $10 reproduction. The Mariner mug is nothing more than a coffee mug decorated to appeal to a boat owner.

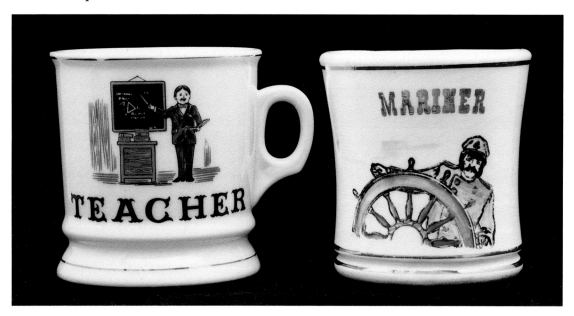

A Japanese import and a coffee mug worth about $10 each.

Dad's Cup.

This is another reproduction variety. They have been around for about twenty years. They can be identified by the letters, "KCI" on the bottom.

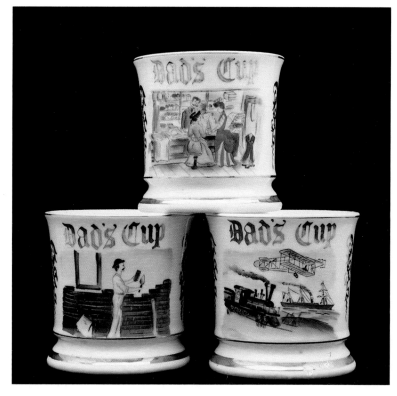

"Dad's Cup" reproductions.

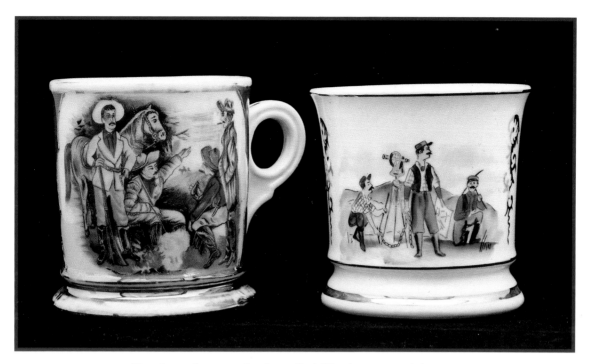

Here is another reproduction called "Cowboys around the Campfire." It is an attractive illustration, but there was no space for a name. The mug to the right is a "Dad's cup" without any wording. It can receive a bogus name and be sold as an Occupational. The reproductions aren't dangerous as long as they can't be personalized.

Fakes

In recent years many fakes have appeared on the collecting scene. These aren't Japanese reproductions with new names, but mugs intended to sell to advanced collectors for thousands of dollars. The people producing these fakes know the mug collecting hobby and they know what type of rare subject matter to place on the mug. The main problem is proving that the mug is fake. If you accuse someone of selling a fake and are unable to prove it, you leave yourself open for legal problems.

As a dealer, I offer a 15 day money back guarantee on any mug that I sell, for any reason. You should ask for the same from any dealer. Someone with a fake may not wish to give you this grace period during which you may determine that the mug is fake.

Let's say you buy a mug from an out of state dealer for $1,000. You determine that the mug is fake once you get home. You call the dealer and he tells you to send the mug back, you do so, but never receive your money back from him. Chasing someone in another state over a thousand dollar debt would be expensive and difficult.

The two safety valves, I would say, to protect you from fakes is never buy a mug for a large amount of money if you have no prior business experience with the dealer. The second is always be aware if a mug looks "too" good. Many fakes that I have seen today have gold letters that are relatively small compared to authentic mugs.

Chapter 5
Barber Bottles

During the era of shaving mugs, barber bottles appeared. These were sold by the distributor to the barber along with large quantities of their tonics and hair oils. The barber could make his own blend and deposit the finished product into his bottles, or he could just pour the supplier's product directly into the bottle.

Most barber bottles are between 7 inches and 10 inches tall. There are two varieties, decorated milk glass and art glass. Much of the art glass was imported from Bohemia, now part of Czechoslovakia. Much of the milk glass was made in the U.S.

Barber bottles were used between 1870 and 1920. During the 1920s the look of the barber shop changed. The concept of "hygienic," often associated with the white garments of the medical profession became the fashion for barbershops too. Many shops got rid of their old look and painted their oak cabinets white and ordered heavy clam broth white barber bottles and accessories to modernize the look of their shops. At this point the old bottles disappeared. However, some barbers still mixed their own potions and put them in the new bottles.

Many of the most desirable barber bottles are the older varieties. These were hand-blown and the glass is very light weight. These also have pontil marks. A pontil was caused when a freshly blown hot bottle was placed on a glass rod which was attached to an iron rod. When the bottle had cooled sufficiently, it was snapped away from the glass rod. This left a round depression about the size of a dime on the bottom of the bottle. It also left a rough surface. In another method the iron rod was curved and the smooth, "improved" pontil was left when it was removed.

As time went on bottles were blown inside of molds and many old bottles don't have pontil marks. During the 1930s barber bottles were made in Mexico. They are much heavier than the Bohemian art glass originals.

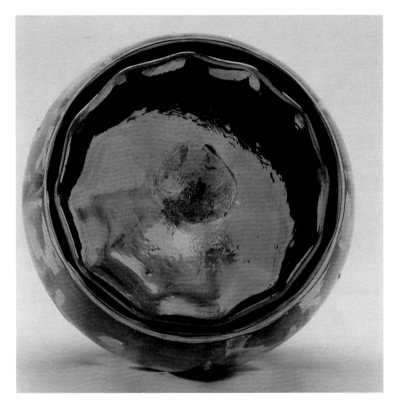

A pontil mark.

Milk glass barber bottles were manufactured to accommodate decoration and a description of bottle contents. Many of them have the same shape, but are of different sizes. The most distinctive bottle was that made by the T. Whitehall Tatum Glass Company of New Jersey. Long before I collected barber bottles I knew of this company as a major manufacturer of telephone insulators. Along with decorations and bottle contents some bottles are personalized and a few denote occupations. T. Whitehall bottles are more valuable with their original metal, screw-top stoppers. Some have a flat top which would accept a regular stopper. They come in two sizes, 8 inch and 10 inch.

Mary Gregory

Some bottles have enamel decorations of children. These are known as "Mary Gregory" glass.

Mary Alice Gregory was born in 1856. As a young woman she lived in Sandwich, Massachusetts She was employed as a veneer decorator, painting decorations for a furniture manufacturer.

In 1880 she was hired by the Boston and Sandwich Glass company to do paintings on lampshades in their decoration department. Mary specialized in landscapes and winter scenes. Her work was considered good, but not distinguishable from the other decorators.

In 1884 she received an inheritance and quit her job. Through frugal living she never had to work again. She died in 1908. She couldn't possibly have imagined that decades after her death she would become famous...for something she never did.

The Sandwich Glass company went out of business in 1888. During the 1920s people began to collect "Sandwich" glass. The interest in Sandwich created an opportunity among antiques dealers. Anything thought to be Sandwich glass had no problem selling. The problem was maintaining a steady inventory. A large number of enameled glass items, showing children at play, began to appear. Collectors were delighted with these items, and they would ask who the artist was.

Mary Gregory never married and lived alone, but she involved herself with church activities in Sandwich. It was known that she had been a decorator in the old glass factory. So when inquiries were made it was her name that the locals remembered.

By the 1930s people who wanted glassware decorated with children asked for Mary Gregory glass. Mary was a lampshade artist and also did some vases, but always landscapes or winter scenes.

Most of the "Mary Gregory" items, including barber bottles, were manufactured in Bohemia and decorated by Bohemian and German artists. Their importation to this country began around 1870. Ten years before Mary worked as a glass decorator.

Label Under Glass

This was a popular and clever process where a paper label or picture was stuck to the back of a thin piece of curved glass and placed over cardboard and glued to the mug or bottle. A similar process was the reverse painting under glass. This is where a name or decoration was painted on the inside of the glass label.

The problem with these was that they couldn't withstand the daily punishment of the barber shop. Soap and water would eat away at the cardboard and glue, and the thin piece of glass was easily cracked or chipped. To find a bottle or mug in perfect condition today is unusual.

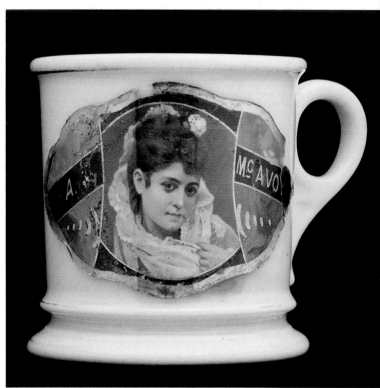

Two label under glass shaving mugs. A similar method was used with barber bottles.

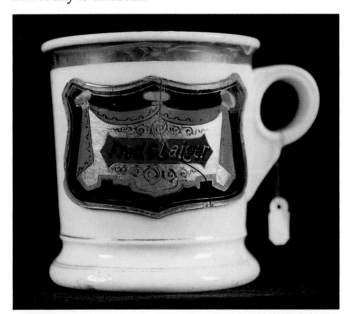

"Tree Bark Covering"

An extremely rare and desirable addition to any mug or bottle collection is a piece with a tree bark covering. This was created using a process combining papier-maché and small twigs. The papier-maché was artistically formed over a glass label bottle or mug and the twigs were cut to look like stumps. Shown here is a bottle and a shaving mug, both items are unusual and difficult to find.

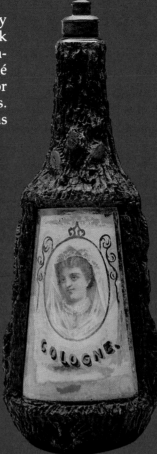

Tree bark bottle with glass label.

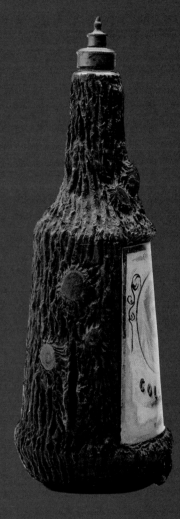

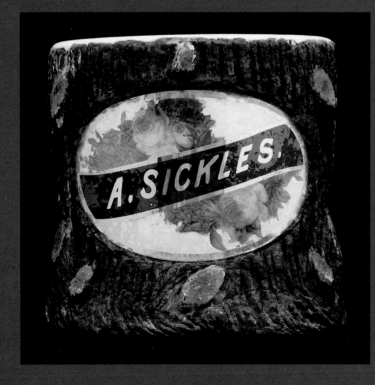

Tree bark shaving mug.

Occupational Bottle, Mug and Bottle Set

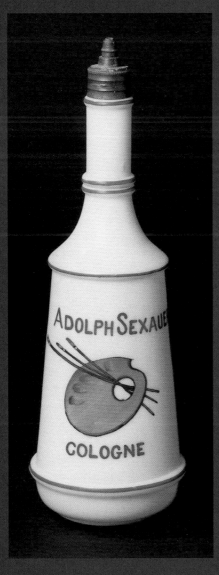

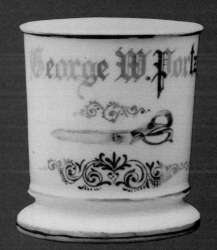

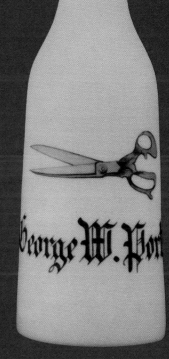

The mug and bottle set is probably the single most difficult item to find in barber shop collectibles. Here we see a fabric cutter's scissors on both the bottle and the mug. I know of about 5 or 6 sets.

Here we see a T. Whitehall Occupational bottle (artist). I only know of a few of these in existence, perhaps twenty.

Brilliantine

Shown here are two Brilliantine bottles next to a standard size barber bottle. Brilliantine was a heavy oil that was used to slick down the customer's hair. It was dispensed in 3" to 3 1/2" bottles. The customer was charged extra for this product. And the small bottle was recognized as the standard dispenser for this special oil.

Brilliantine bottles are hard to find. The two examples shown are priced between $100-200. They should sell for more, but most bottle collectors like standard size items for their collection. The catalog insert shows a Brilliantine bottle for sale.

Two Brilliantine bottles next on either side of a standard barber bottle.

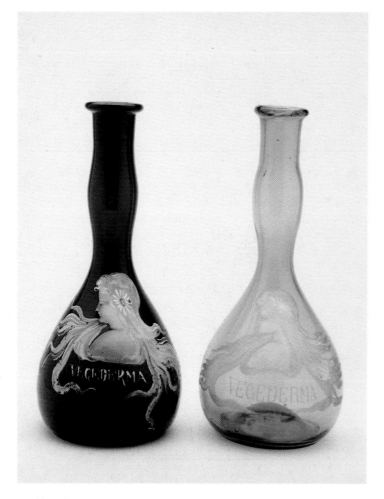

Vegederma bottles.

Vegederma

Vegederma was a popular perfumed hair tonic. The barber could buy a gallon from the distributor for about $4. The special bottles were used to insure the customer that he was getting this particular product. The bottles all have the same enamel design, a girl with flowing hair and the word "Vegederma." Bottles in cobalt and amethyst are the common examples. Vegederma bottles sell for $250-$350.

At the right are three pages from the Holtzhauer Catalog. Note that this catalog refers to shaving paper "urns," most catalogs use the term "vase."

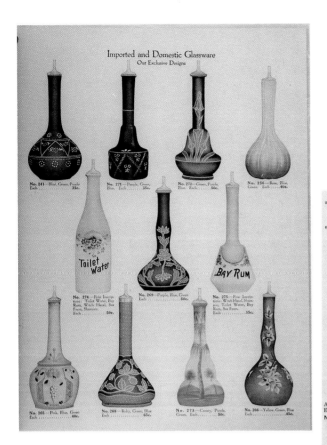

Imported and Domestic Glassware
Our Exclusive Designs

No. 241—Blue, Green, Purple Each..........35c.

No. 271—Purple, Green, Blue. Each.......35c.

No. 272—Green, Purple, Blue. Each......50c.

No. 256—Rose, Blue, Green. Each.......40c.

No. 274—Plain Inscriptions: Toilet Water, Bay Rum, Witch Hazel, Sea Foam, Shampoo. Each.......50c.

No. 269—Purple, Blue, Green. Each.......50c.

No. 275—Fine Inscriptions: Witch Hazel, Shampoo, Toilet Water, Bay Rum, Sea Foam. Each...........55c.

No. 265—Pink, Blue, Green Each.........40c.

No. 268—Ruby, Green, Blue Each..........65c.

No. 273—Canary, Purple, Green. Each.......50c.

No. 266—Yellow, Green, Blue Each...........45c.

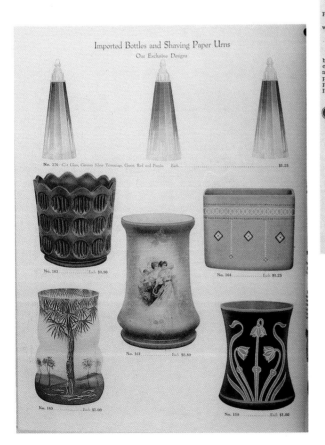

Imported Bottles and Shaving Paper Urns
Our Exclusive Designs

No. 276—Cut Glass, Green Silver Trimmings, Green, Red and Purple. Each...........$1.25

No. 163..........Each $0.50

No. 164...........Each $1.25

No. 161...........Each $0.80

No. 165..........Each $1.00

No. 159..........Each $1.00

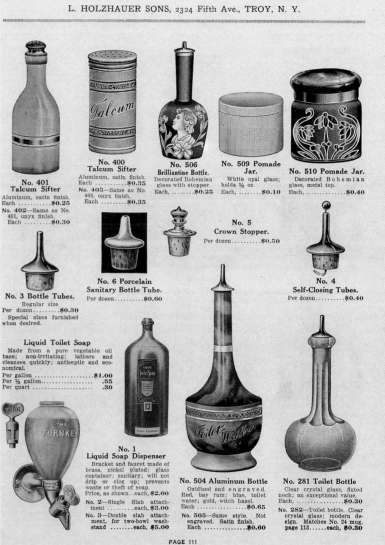

No. 401 Talcum Sifter
Aluminum, satin finish. Each..........$0.25
No. 402—Same as No. 401, onyx finish. Each........$0.30

No. 400 Talcum Sifter
Aluminum, satin finish. Each...........$0.35
No. 403—Same as No. 400, onyx finish. Each........$0.35

No. 506 Brilliantine Bottle.
Decorated Bohemian glass with stopper. Each,........$0.25

No. 509 Pomade Jar.
White opal glass; holds ½ oz. Each,.......$0.10

No. 510 Pomade Jar.
Decorated Bohemian glass, metal top. Each,..............$0.40

No. 5 Crown Stopper.
Per dozen..........$0.50

No. 3 Bottle Tubes.
Regular size
Per dozen.........$0.30
Special sizes furnished when desired.

No. 6 Porcelain Sanitary Bottle Tube.
Per dozen..........$0.60

No. 4 Self-Closing Tubes.
Per dozen..........$0.40

Liquid Toilet Soap
Made from a pure vegetable oil base; non-irritating; lathers and cleanses quickly; antiseptic and economical.
Per gallon $1.00
Per ½ gallon.................. .55
Per quart .... .30

No. 1 Liquid Soap Dispenser
Bracket and faucet made of brass, nickel plated; glass container; sanitary; will not drip or clog up; prevents waste or theft of soap.
Price, as shown..each, $2.00
No. 2—Single slab attachment ....each, $3.00
No. 3—Double slab attachment, for two-bowl washstand ....each, $5.00

No. 504 Aluminum Bottle
Oxidized and engraved. Red, bay rum; blue, toilet water; gold, witch hazel. Each $0.65
No. 505—Same style. Not engraved. Satin finish. Each $0.60

No. 281 Toilet Bottle
Clear crystal glass; fluted neck; an exceptional value. Each, ...$0.30
No. 282—Toilet bottle. Clear crystal glass; modern design. Matches No. 24 mug, page 113......each, $0.30

PAGE 111

From the Holzhauer Catalog

193

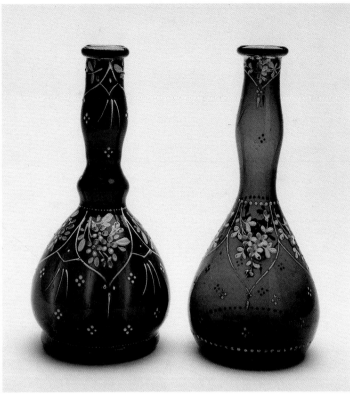

Left, cobalt with floral enamel. Right, green floral enamel.

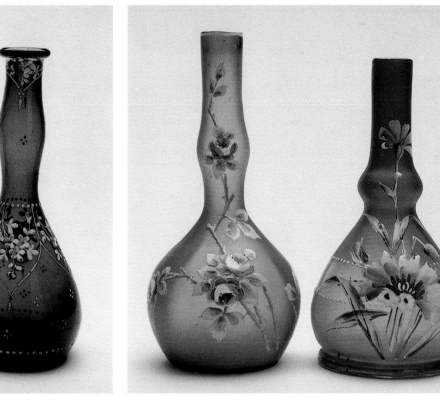

Left, frosted honey amber with rose decoration. Right, frosted red and pink with floral design.

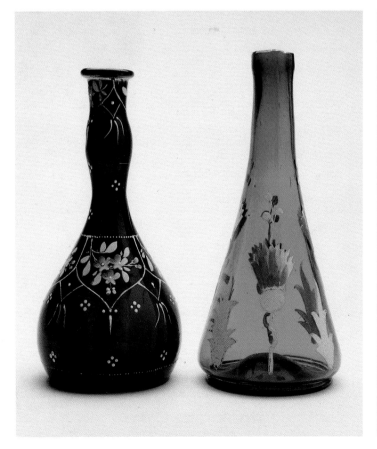

Left, amethyst with floral enamel. Right, green with thistle decoration.

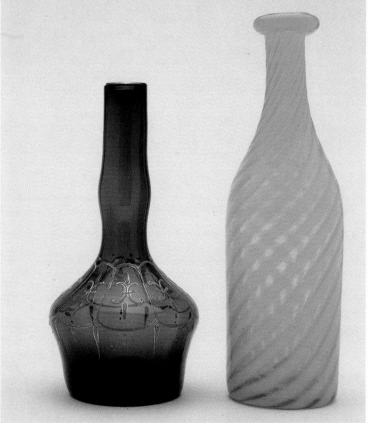

Left, amethyst with gold decoration. Right, opalized blue swirl.

Shaving paper vase

Another art glass item that is not well known is the shaving paper vase. This was a container that held the used tissue paper which wiped the whiskers and shaving soap from the razor. These items usually could be ordered with the same design as certain barber bottles. Because these items were large they didn't have the same appeal as mugs or bottles. Conse-quently very few survive today. Shaving paper vases are 8 to 10 inches tall and are 5 inches across.

Except for a few examples, the barber bottle and shaving paper vase collection shown here is that of Mr. Anthony Gugliotti. Perhaps the finest collection known.

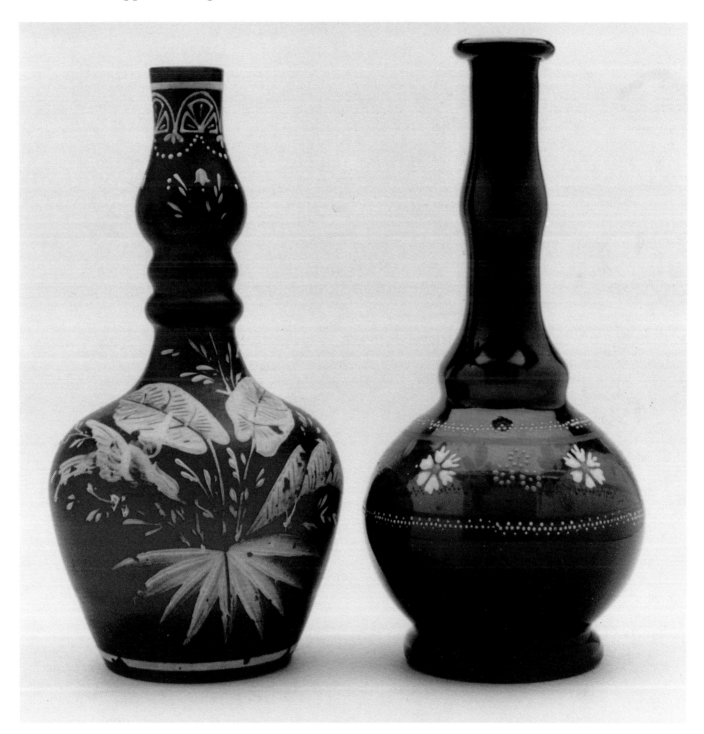

Left, frosted cobalt with cream enamel. Right, amethyst with small decoration.

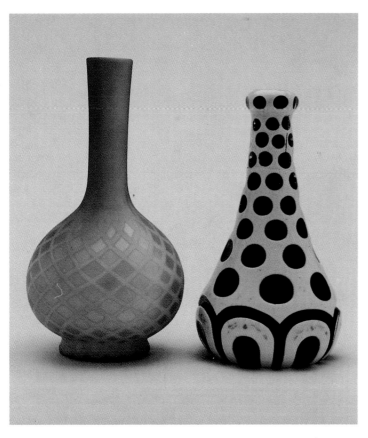

Left, coral satin quilt pattern. Right, dark green with white cut overlay.

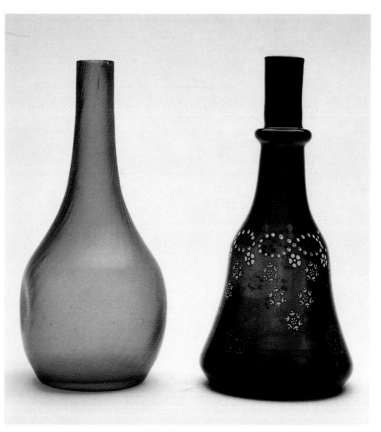

Left, amber "pinched" type. Right, green bell shape.

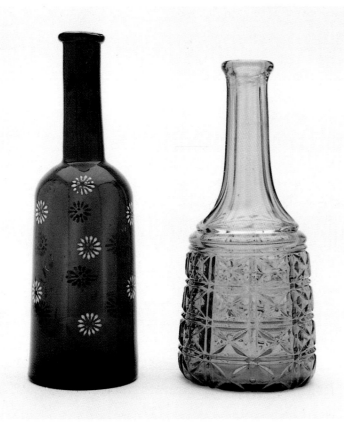

Left, cobalt with floral. Right, blue flint glass.

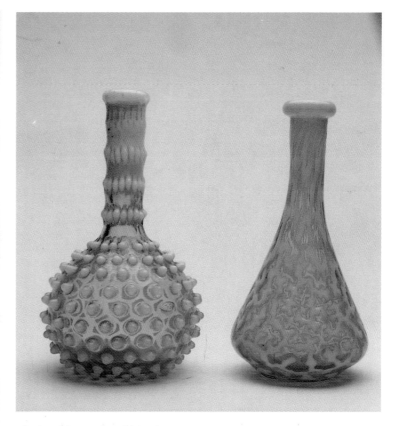

Left, white opalized blue hobnail. Right, blue Spanish Lace, opalized.

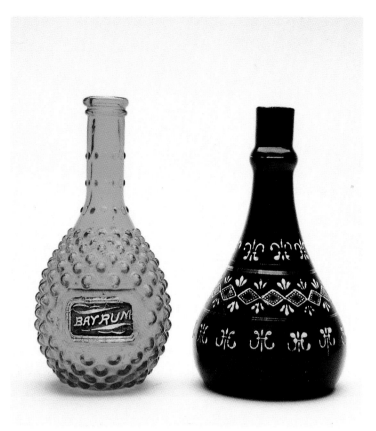

Left, blue hobnail, label under glass. Right, amethyst, white enamelled with gold.

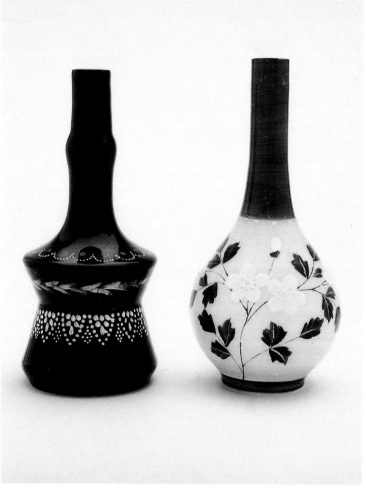

Left, amethyst enamel decoration. Right, milk glass with floral painting.

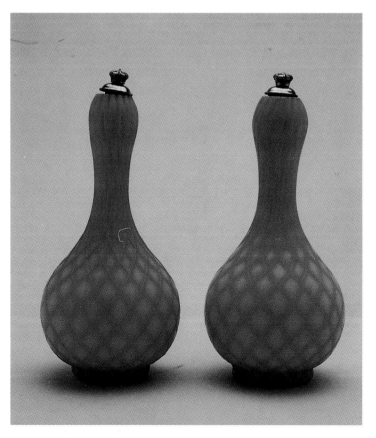

Set, green satin quilt pattern.

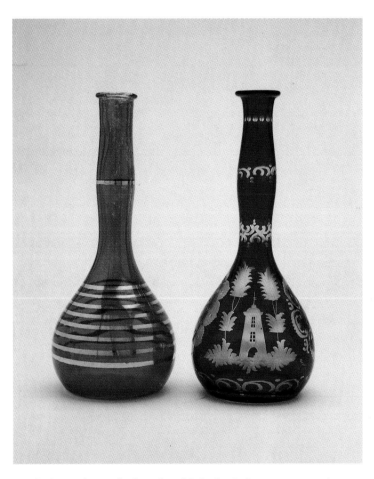

Left, cranberry flash with gold. Right, Bohemian, cut to clear.

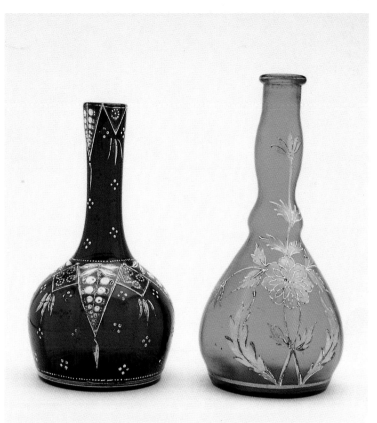

Left, cobalt, heavily enamelled. Right, light blue, gold floral design.

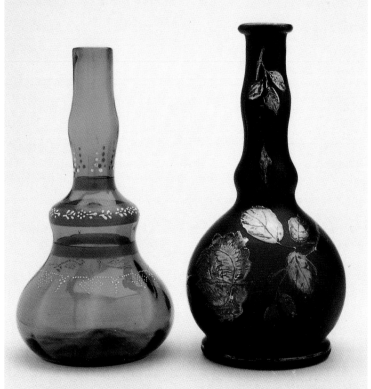

Left, teal blue with enamelled decoration. Right, Amethyst, satin with silver overlay.

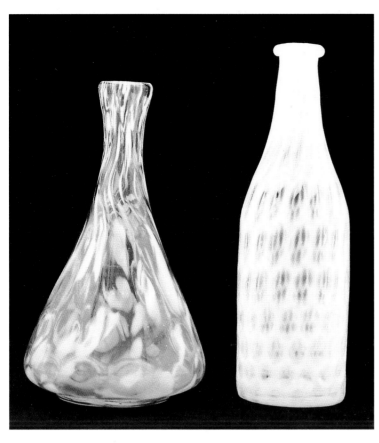

Left, yellow-green end of day. Right, light lime yellow, thumbprint.

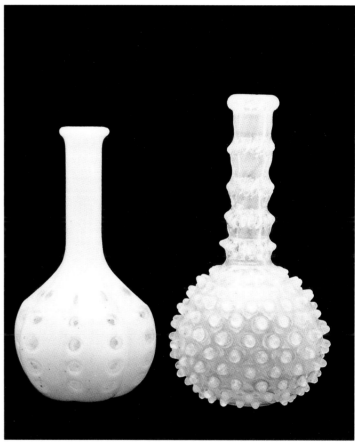

Left, white opalized, coin spot. Right, white opalized hobnail.

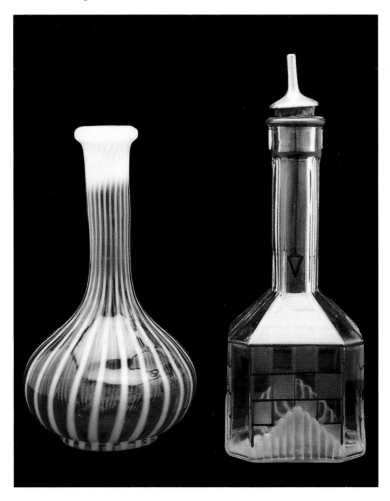

Left, candy stripe, white opalized. Right, rare art deco type.

199

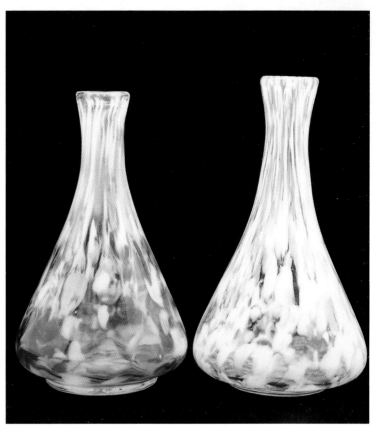

Left, light blue, end of day thumbprint. Right, orange, end of day.

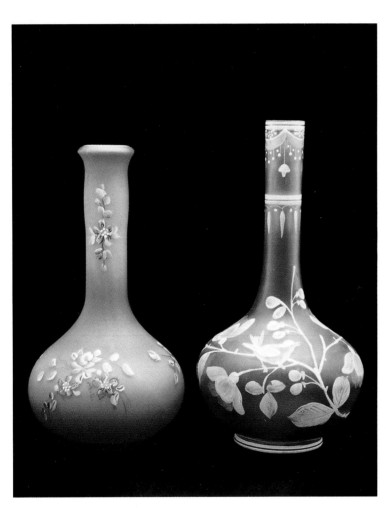

Left, red satin case glass. Right, honey-amber satin with white decoration.

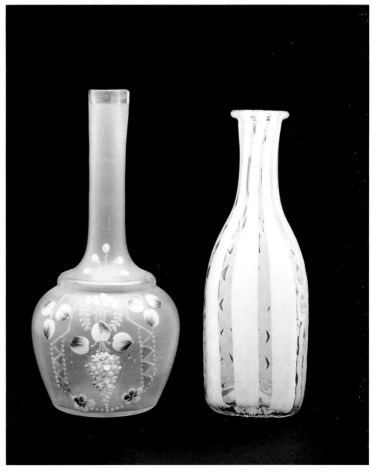

Left, light blue satin with embossed grape design. Right, clear, with white encased bands.

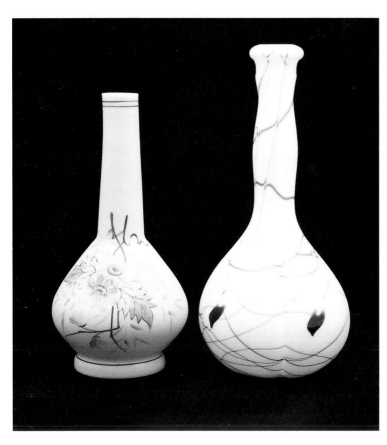

Left, pink decorated milk glass. Right, Fenton glass, ivory with brown design.

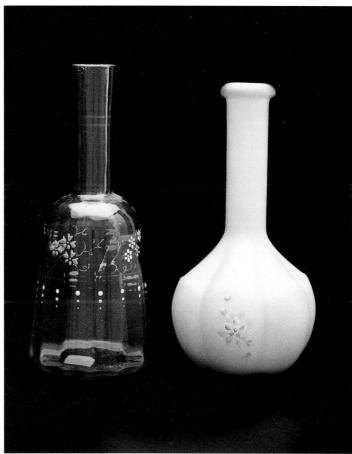

Left, light amber with enamel. Right, satin case glass, melon shape.

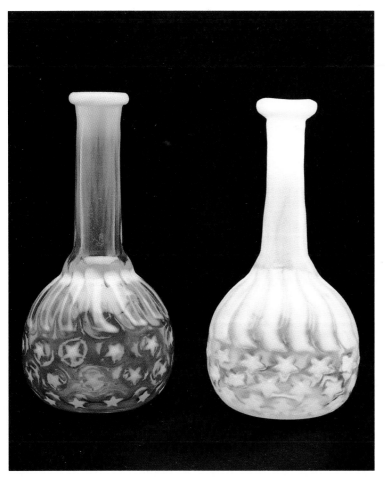

Left, blue stars and stripes pattern. Right, white stars and stripes.

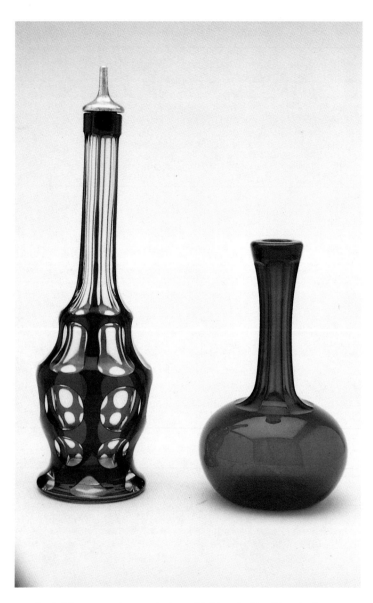

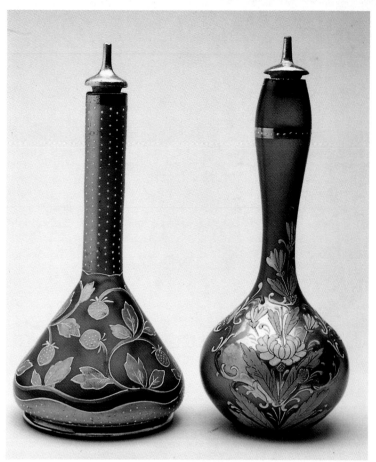

Left, green satin with strawberries. Right, green satin with gold and enamelled design.

Left, blue over clear out glass. Right, cobalt with cut glass neck.

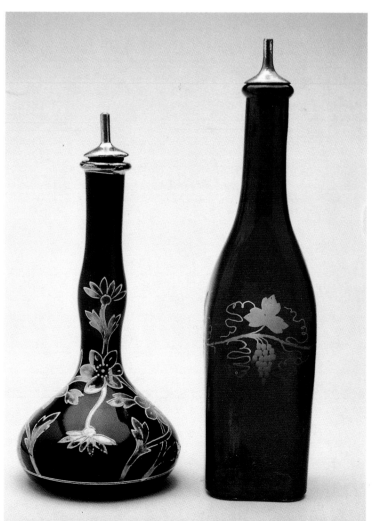

Left, amethyst with gold floral decoration. Right, cranberry cut to clear.

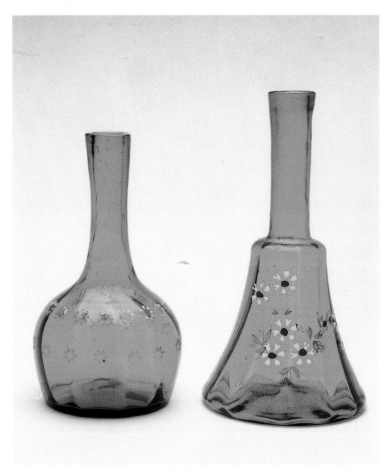

Left, teal blue with small enamelled design. Right, teal blue bell shaped.

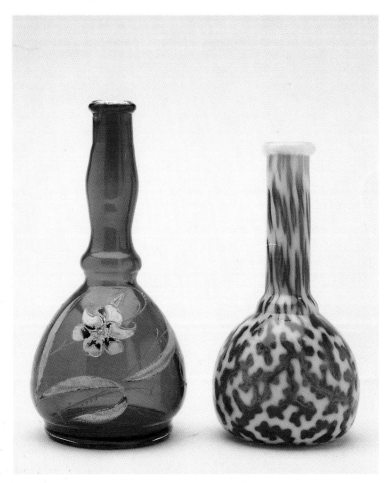

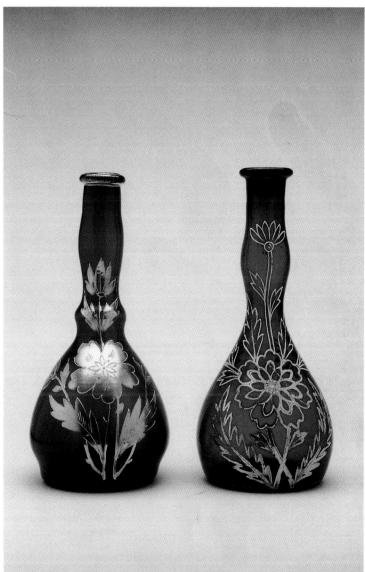

Left, amethyst, satin with gold floral design. Right, emerald with gold floral design.

Left, red with enamelled floral design. Right, red opalized spanish lace.

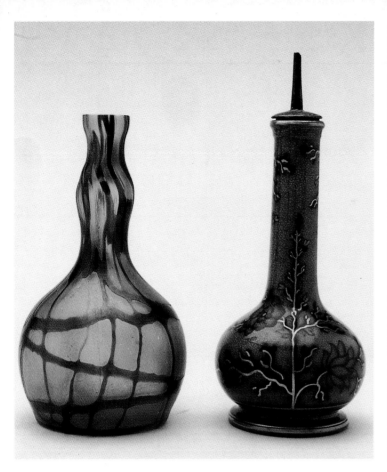

Left, Lotz type art glass. Right, glazed pottery.

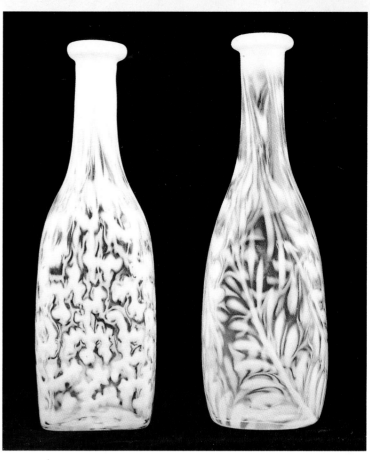

Left, opalized spanish lace. Right, opalized fern pattern.

Left, red case glass with gold design. Right, clear over yellow case glass, quilt pattern.

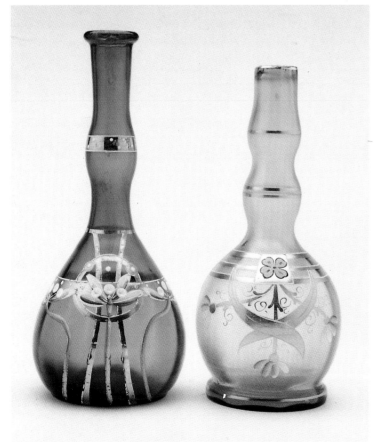

Left, blue satin with gold and enamel. Right, light green satin.

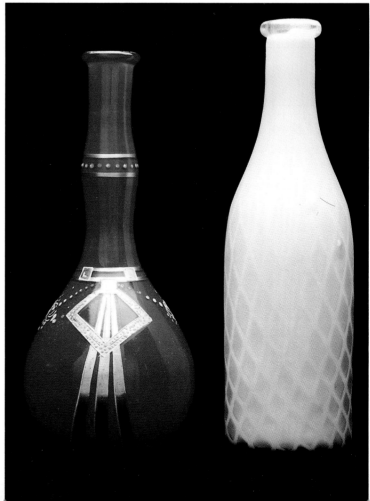

Left, cranberry with white swirl. Right, tall bottle, cranberry with white swirl.

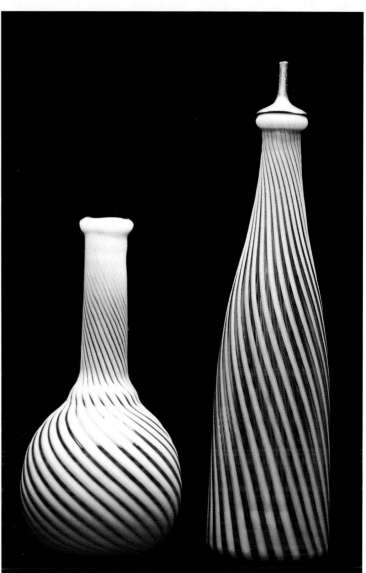

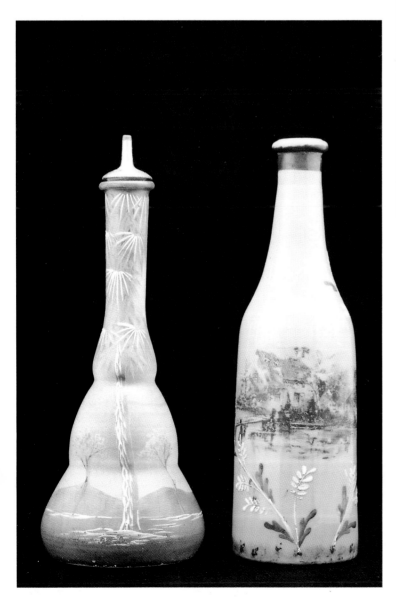

Left, green frosted palm tree design. Right, blue birds egg color with design.

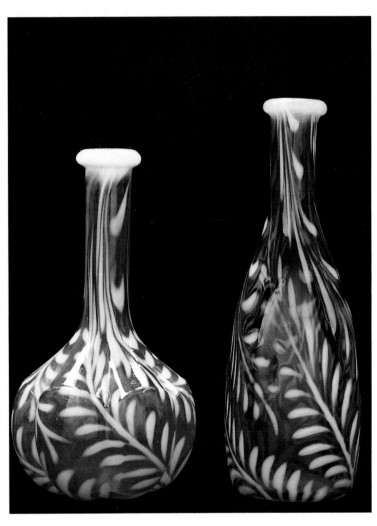

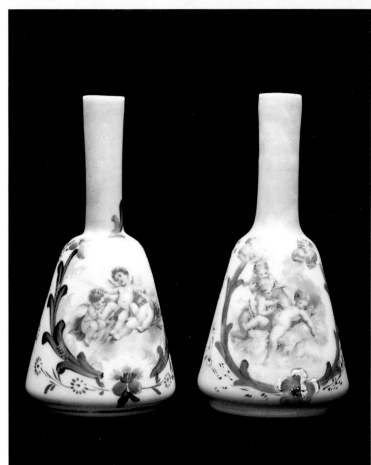

Left and right, milk glass decorated with cherubs, two different designs.

Left, cranberry opalized fern, melon shape. Right, cranberry opalized fern, straight bottle.

Left, opalized cranberry. Right, green thumbprint.

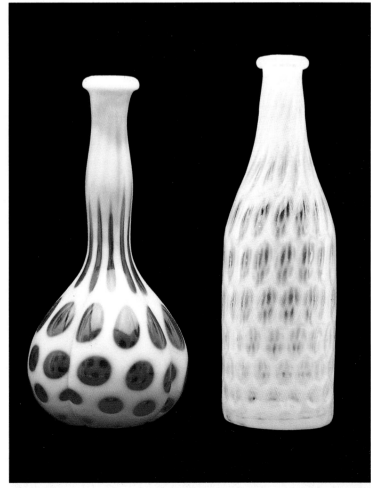

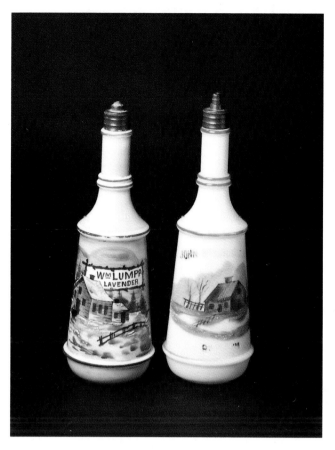

Left, personalized "Lavender". Right, winter scene, name worn. *Courtesy of Thomas and Penelope Nader.*

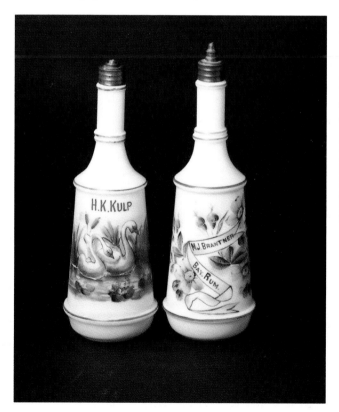

Left, personalized "swans". Right, personalized "Bay Rum".
Courtesy of Thomas and Penelope Nader.

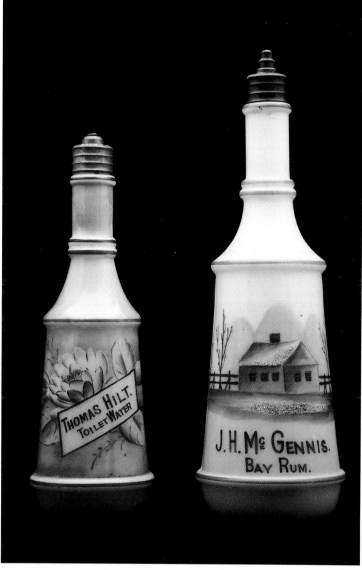

Left, small size 8", personalized "toilet water". Right, large size 10", personalized "Bay Rum". *Anthony Gugliotti.*

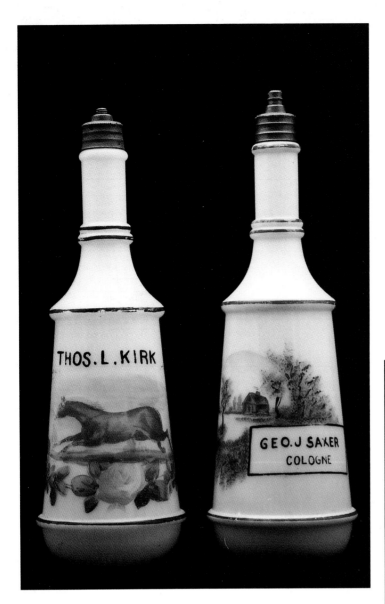

Left, horse decorative, personalized. Right, personalized "cologne". *Anthony Gugliotti.*

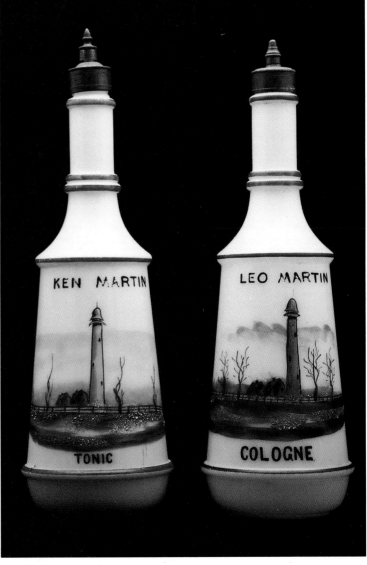

Left, personalized "Lighthouse" design. Right, same, probably a set made for brothers.

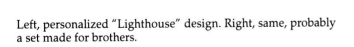

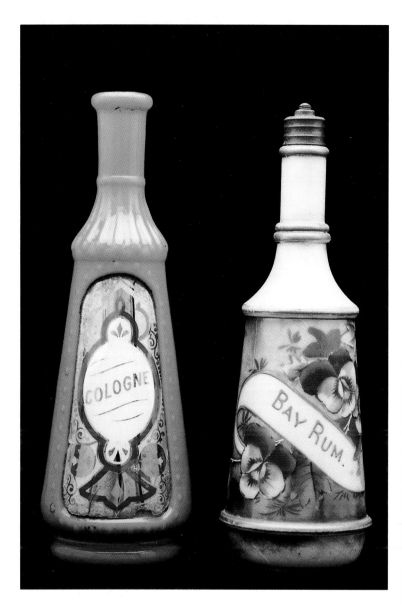

Left, blue milk glass, large reverse painting under glass. Right, T. Whitehall, pansy decor, "Bay Rum". *Anthony Gugliotti.*

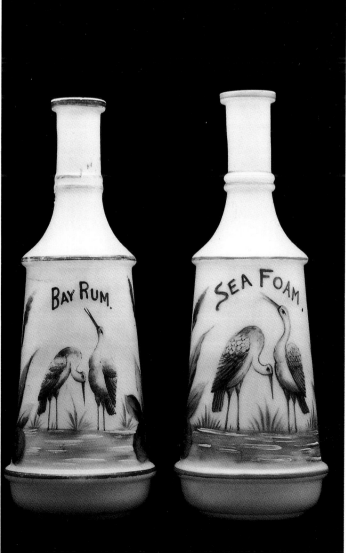

Set, flat top T. Whitehall, "Cormorant" design, non-personalized. *Anthony Gugliotti.*

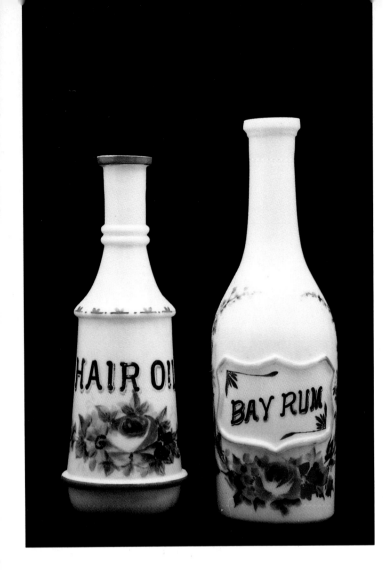

Left, flat top, hair oil, 8", T. Whitehall. Right, bay rum in shield raised design. *Anthony Gugliotti.*

Set, tulip design milk glass. *Anthony Gugliotti.*

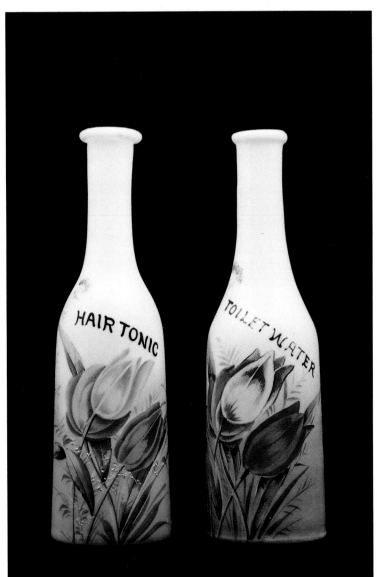

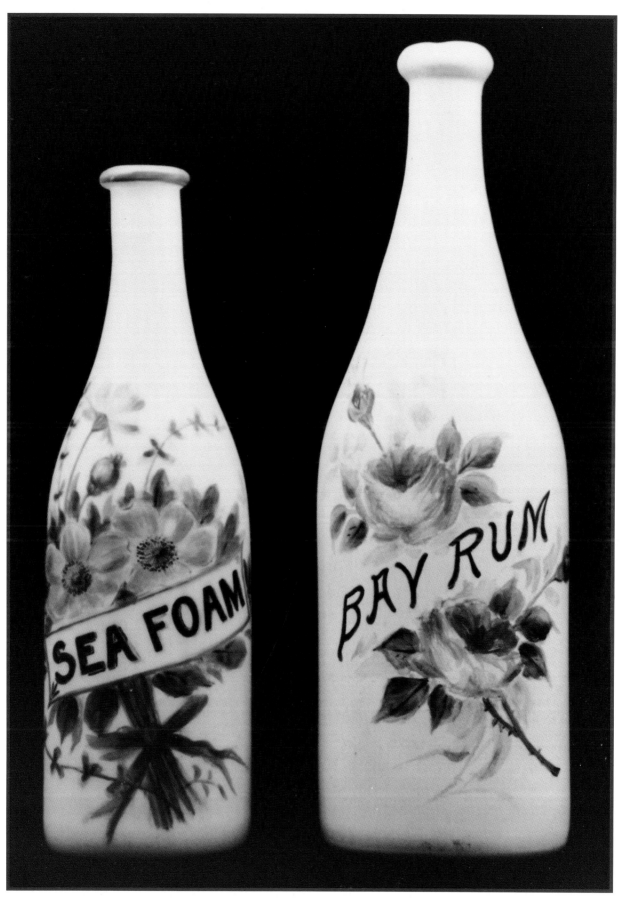

Left, floral with "sea foam". Right, quart size, roses with "Bay Rum". *Anthony Gugliotti.*

Left, floral "toilet water". Right, floral sea foam. *Anthony Gugliotti.*

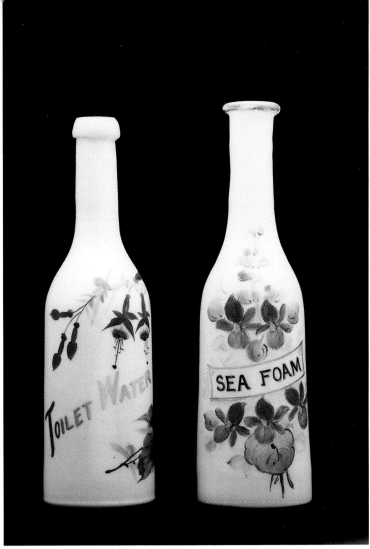

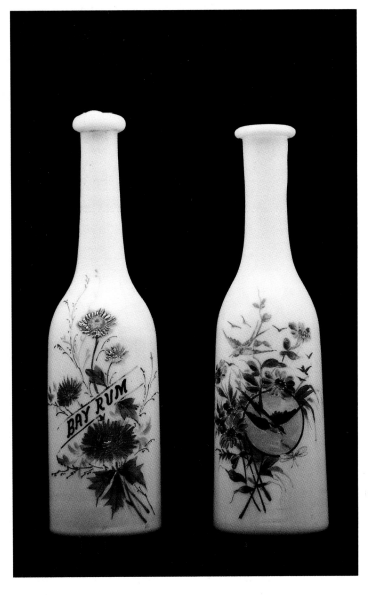

Left, floral "Bay Rum". Right, moon and bird decoration. *Anthony Gugliotti.*

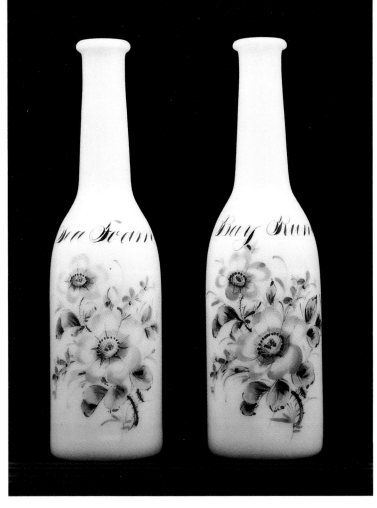

Set, floral decorated "Sea foam" and "Bay Rum". *Anthony Gugliotti.*

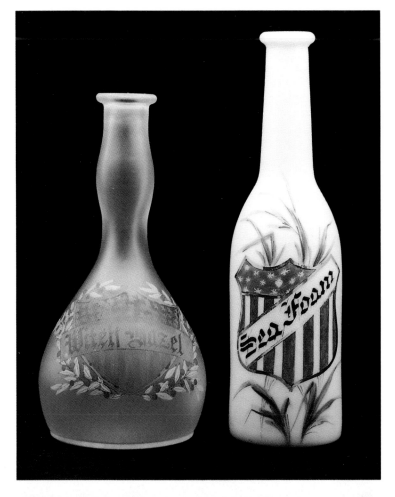

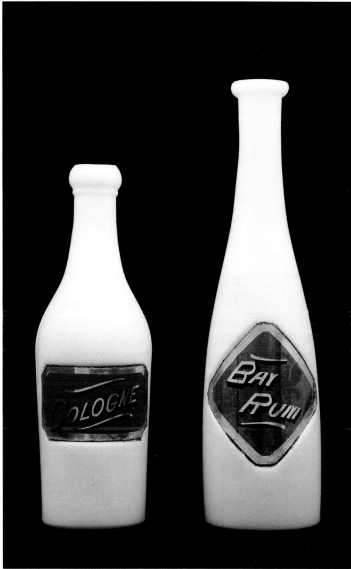

Left, "Cologne" reverse painting under glass. Right, "Bay Rum" reverse painting under glass. *Anthony Gugliotti.*

Left, American shield over clear frosted glass. Right, shield design, on milk glass. *Anthony Gugliotti.*

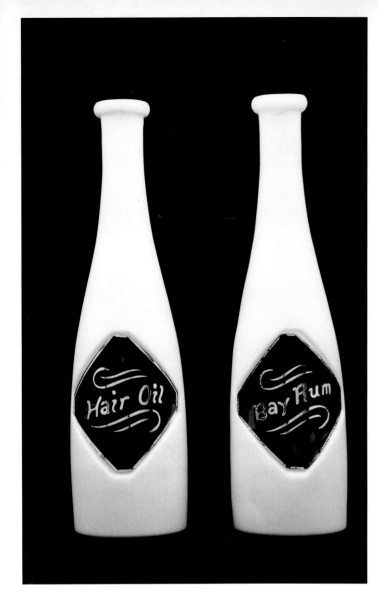

Set, white milk glass, label under glass. *Anthony Gugliotti.*

Set, reverse painting under glass. *Anthony Gugliotti.*

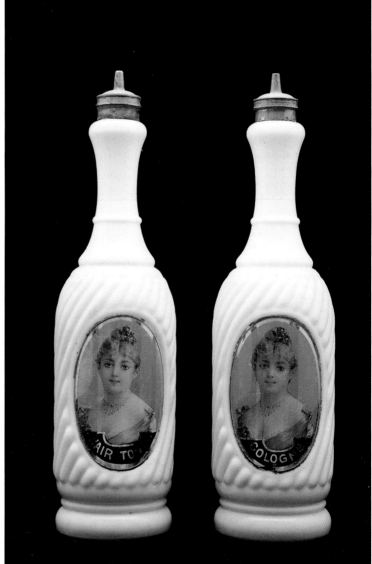

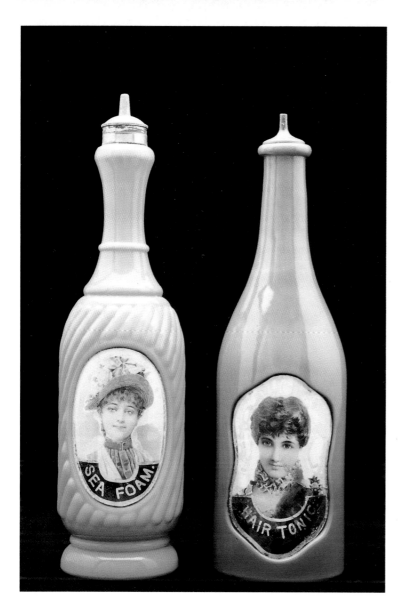

Left, sea foam, blue milk glass, perfect. Right, "Quart" shape, dark blue, unusual. *Anthony Gugliotti.*

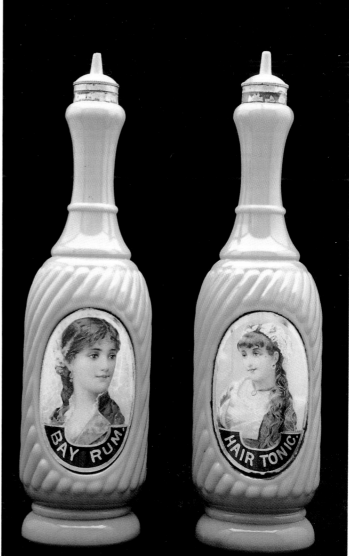

Left, blue milk glass, perfect. Right, blue milk glass, perfect. *Anthony Gugliotti.*

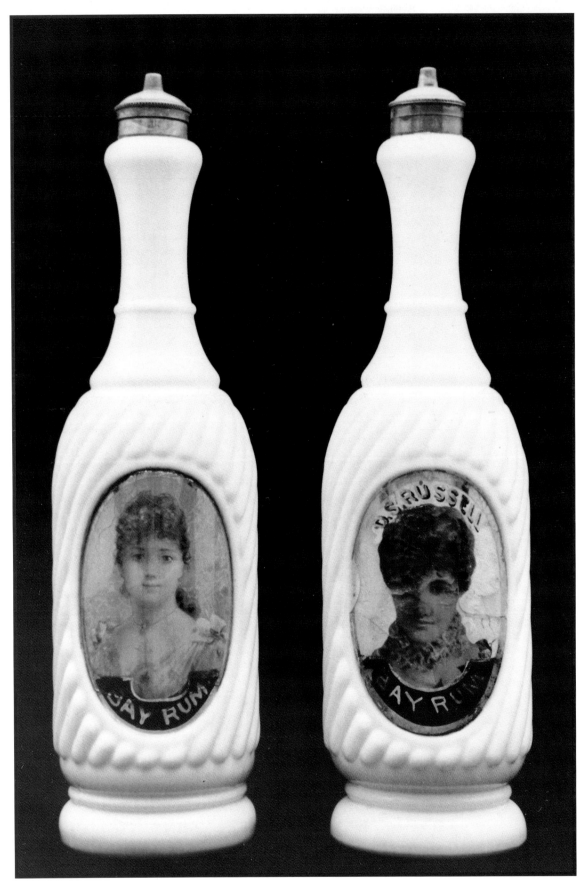

Left, Bay Rum, slight damage, white milk glass. Right, personalized "Bay Rum", white milk glass, serious damage. *Anthony Gugliotti.*

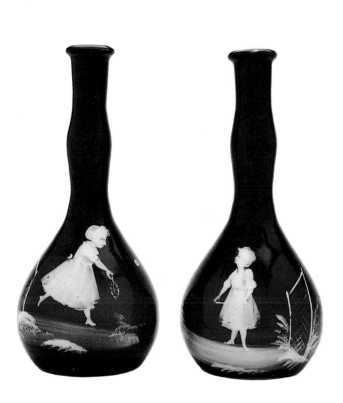

Left, cobalt, tennis design. Right, cobalt, tennis design.

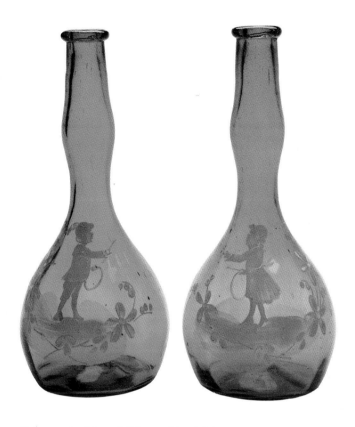

Set, powder blue, children with stick hoops.

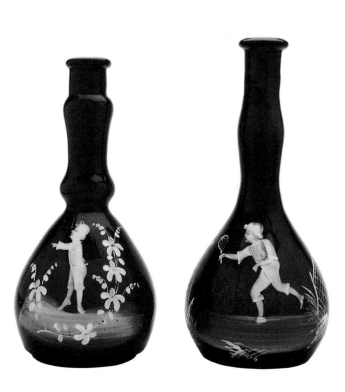

Left, cobalt, child with flowers. Right, cobalt, tennis design.

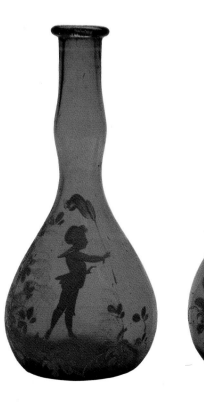

Set, green, children with butterfly nets.

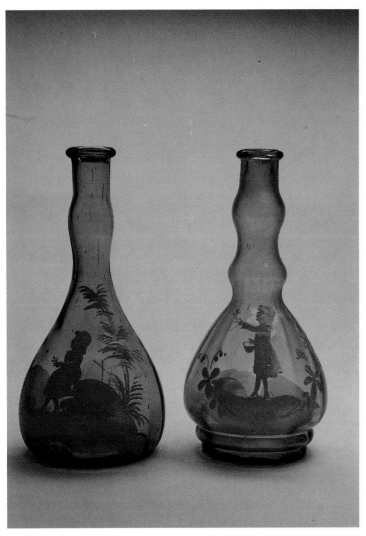

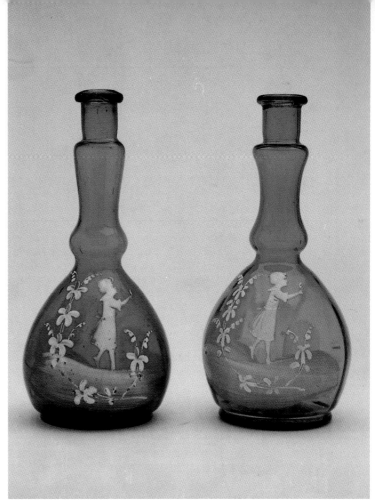

Set, emerald green, children with flowers.

Left, yellow-green, child on rock. Right, light green, child picking flowers.

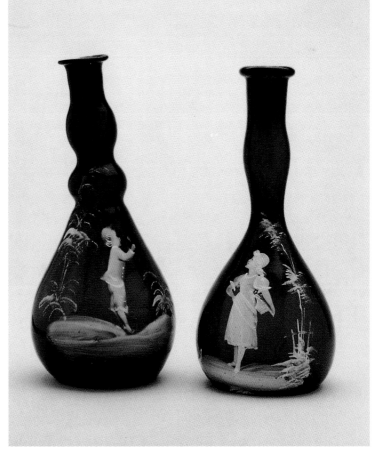

Left, amethyst, bent neck. Right, amethyst, girl with basket.

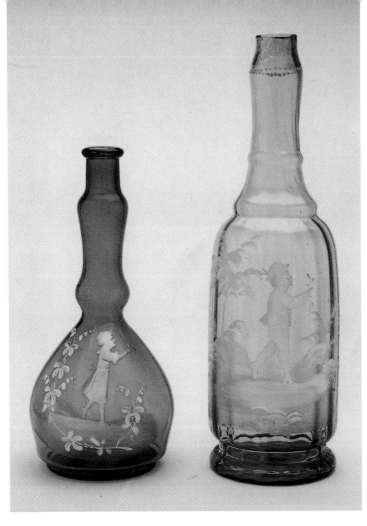

Left, teal blue, child with floral design. Right, light smokey amber, tall bottle with large design.

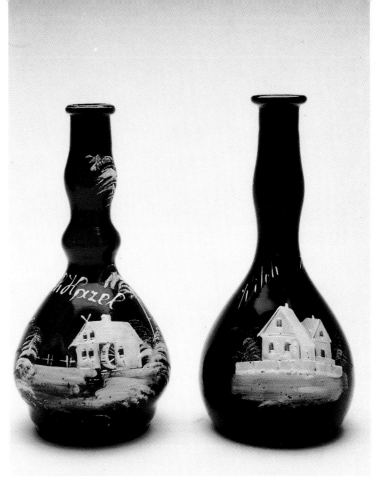

Left, amethyst, grist mill "Witch Hazel". Right, amethyst, house with wall, "Witch Hazel".

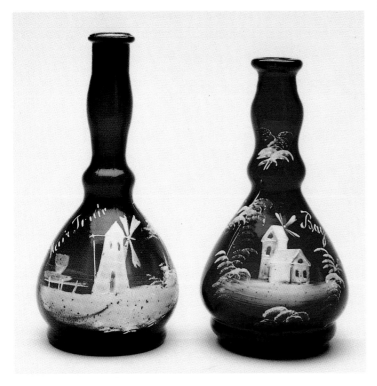

Windmill design, left, amethyst with "Hair Tonic". Right, cobalt with "Bay Rum".

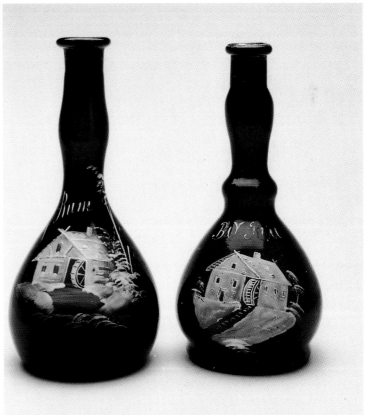

Amethyst, both "Bay Rum" with grist mill design.

219

Shaving paper vase

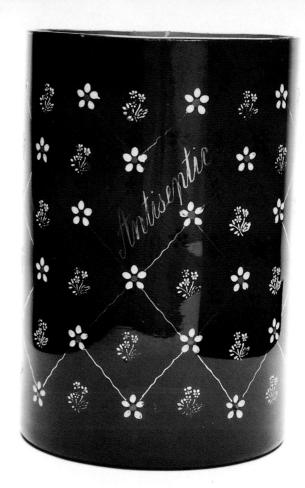

Amethyst with enamelled decoration and "Antiseptic" in gold. *Courtesy of Anthony Gugliotti.*

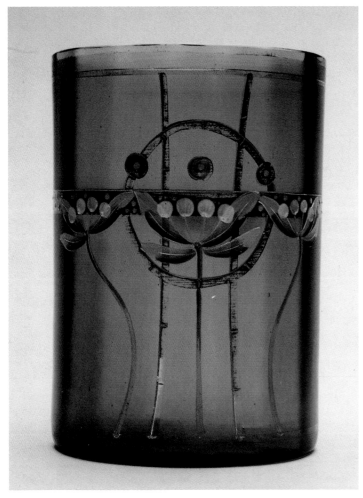

Satin blue with enamel decoration. *Courtesy of Anthony Gugliotti.*

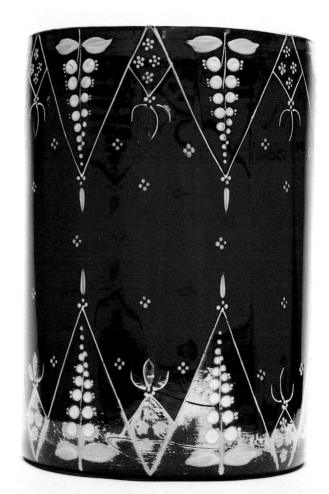

Cobalt with ivory enamel decoration. *Courtesy of Anthony Gugliotti.*

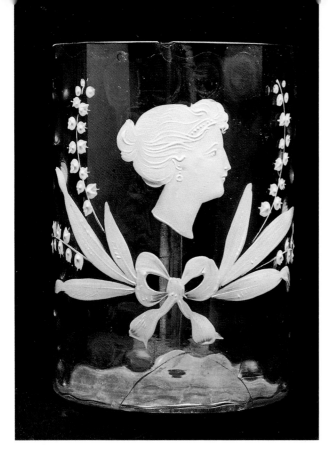

Amber-Orange, thumbprint, with cameo style enamelled design. *Courtesy of Anthony Gugliotti.*

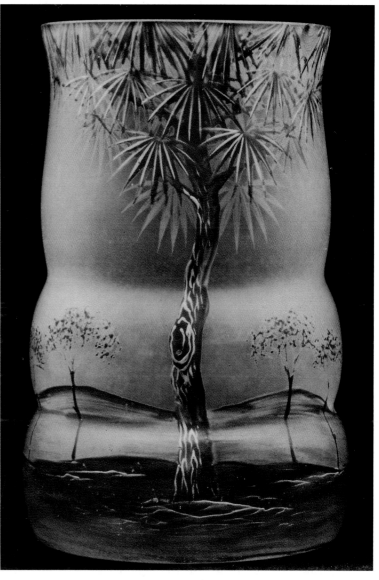

Frosted clear with red palm tree design, as shown in the catalog. *Courtesy of Anthony Gugliotti.*

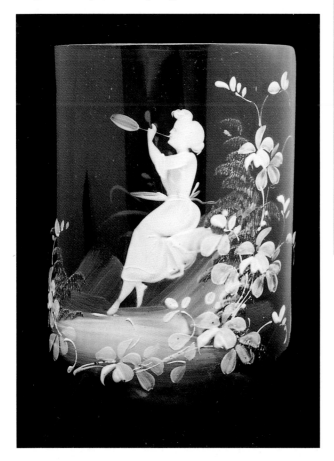

Dark green with "Mary Gregory" design. *Courtesy of Anthony Gugliotti.*

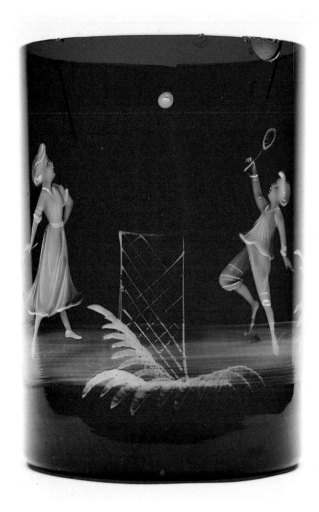

Cobalt, "Mary Gregory" tennis design, the most commonly found. *Courtesy of Anthony Gugliotti.*

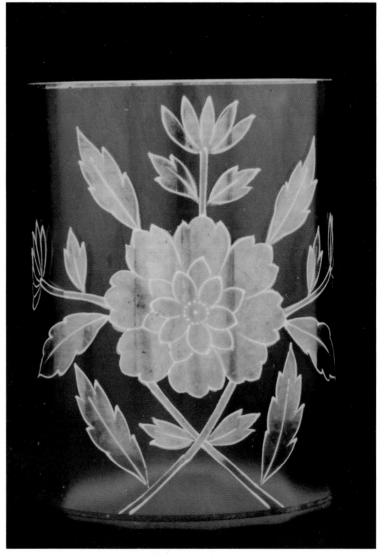

Green satin with gold floral finish. *Courtesy of Anthony Gugliotti.*

Chapter 6
Other Barber Shop Collectibles

Advertising

The barber shop, like any other retail business, would advertise items and services it wished to sell. The supplier's helped the barber by providing him with various forms of display material, designed to attract the eye of the customer.

Mug Sheets

Mug sheets were designed to hang on the shop wall. They came in various sizes and in black and white or color. Some just featured mugs while others had combinations of retail items.

The sheet shown here is from the T. Noonan and Sons of Boston. It has mugs with prices (mug sheets had the barber's profit included in the price).

I would say that 98% of mug sheets were destroyed. They would have been thrown out after the mug era or sooner if the mug prices changed. Catalogs had a better chance of being saved, as they contained other supplies and equipment the barber would need for his shop.

One mug sheet that is rather common is that of "B. Stuebner's and Sons" of Brooklyn, New York. Because of the large number of perfect condition sheets, I think these were factory extras which were never distributed. It is a rather small sheet and it is not in color.

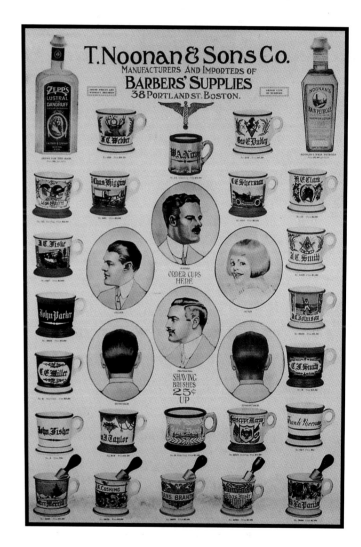

This sheet has everything you would want in an early advertising item: large size, 30" x 20"; illustrations in color; and outstanding condition, the most difficult feature to find.

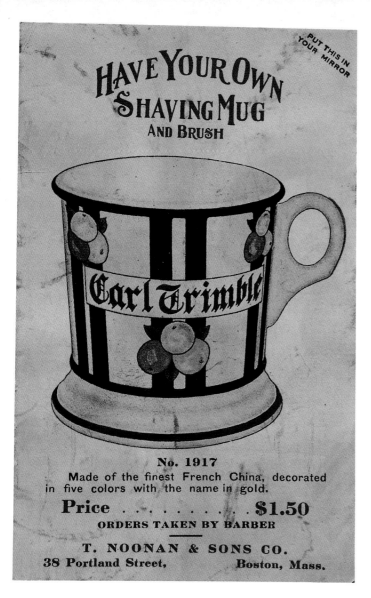

A Noonan mirror card.

Mirror Cards

Another advertising gimmick was the mirror card. This was meant to fit between the barber's mirror and its wooden frame. These could be placed at eye level for the customer. The example shown, which is from Noonan's, is 3 1/2" x 5". These are hard to find, color and condition are always positive factors.

Advertising Mugs and Bottles

After a shave or haircut the customer could select from a variety of head rubs or facial splashes. The barber could sell these for a small extra charge or it could be included in the standard price.

Many of these items would be sold by the bottle. Shown here are several unused labels from retail items of P. Eisemann. Mr. Eisemann was a barber, barber supplier, and a shaving mug decorator.

Some bottles have ornate labels and others have labels under glass. They are sought by certain collectors.

A few suppliers produced mugs and bottles as give-aways to promote a new product line, such as shaving soap or tonic. These items usually sell for under $100.

Labels from Phil Eisemann's products.

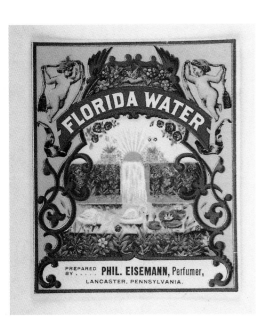

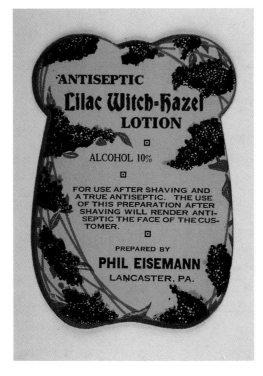

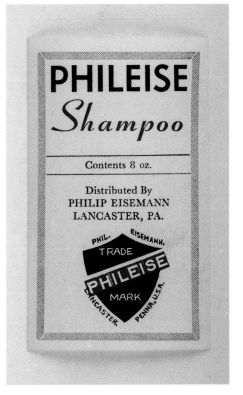

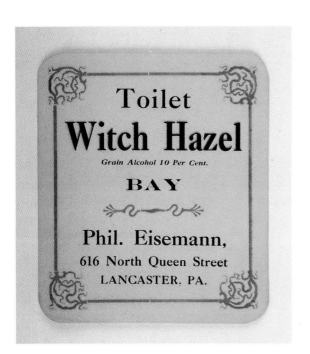

Toilet
Witch Hazel
Grain Alcohol 10 Per Cent.

BAY

Phil. Eisemann,
616 North Queen Street
LANCASTER, PA.

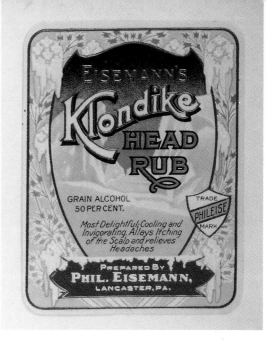

EISEMANN'S
Klondike
HEAD RUB

GRAIN ALCOHOL
50 PER CENT.

TRADE PHILEISE MARK

Most Delightful, Cooling and Invigorating, Allays Itching of the Scalp and relieves Headaches

PREPARED BY
PHIL. EISEMANN,
LANCASTER, PA.

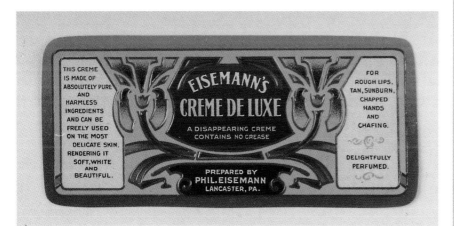

THIS CREME IS MADE OF ABSOLUTELY PURE AND HARMLESS INGREDIENTS AND CAN BE FREELY USED ON THE MOST DELICATE SKIN, RENDERING IT SOFT, WHITE AND BEAUTIFUL.

EISEMANN'S
CREME DE LUXE
A DISAPPEARING CREME
CONTAINS NO GREASE

FOR ROUGH LIPS, TAN, SUNBURN, CHAPPED HANDS AND CHAFING.

DELIGHTFULLY PERFUMED.

PREPARED BY
PHIL. EISEMANN,
LANCASTER, PA.

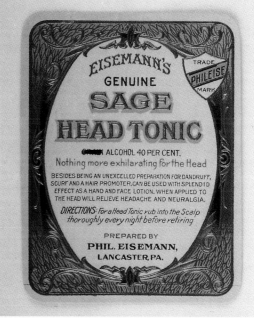

EISEMANN'S
GENUINE
SAGE
HEAD TONIC

TRADE PHILEISE MARK

ALCOHOL 40 PER CENT.
Nothing more exhilarating for the Head

BESIDES BEING AN UNEXCELLED PREPARATION FOR DANDRUFF, SCURF AND A HAIR PROMOTER, CAN BE USED WITH SPLENDID EFFECT AS A HAND AND FACE LOTION. WHEN APPLIED TO THE HEAD WILL RELIEVE HEADACHE AND NEURALGIA.

DIRECTIONS: *for a Head Tonic rub into the Scalp thoroughly every night before retiring*

PREPARED BY
PHIL. EISEMANN,
LANCASTER, PA.

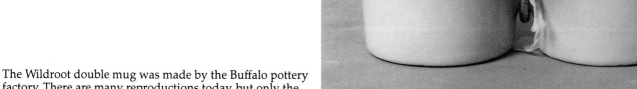

The Wildroot double mug was made by the Buffalo pottery factory. There are many reproductions today, but only the originals carry the Buffalo mark.

225

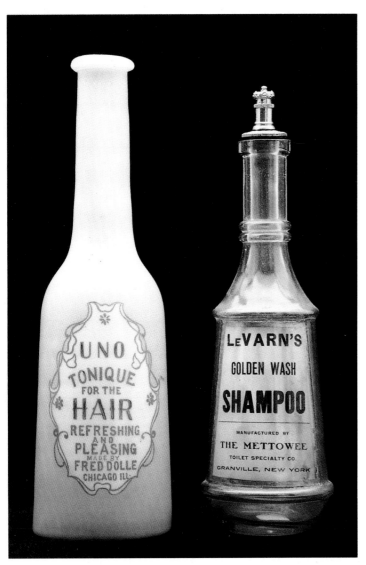

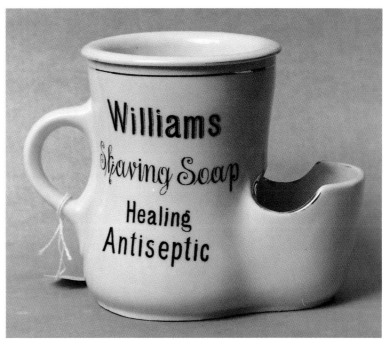

Giveaway mugs to promote shaving soaps.

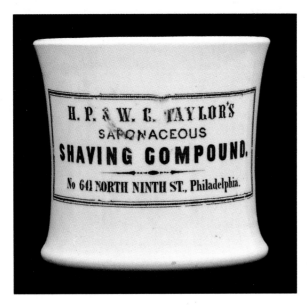

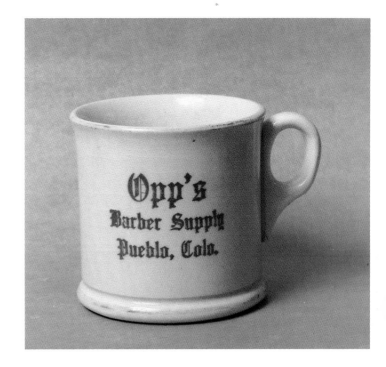

226

Photographs

In recent years mug collectors have started to collect photos of old barber shops. For many years photograph collectors have sought these as well. Their collecting interest lies with working shops of a hundred years ago. Interiors of businesses such as butcher shops, police stations and dry goods stores are preferred.

Mug collectors wishing to collect barber shop photos should keep a few considerations in mind.

Always try to find pictures that are clear and show many details, such as advertising, views of mug racks, dated material like calendars, shoe shine stand and other unique items. Shown here are two examples of barber shop interiors.

The down side of photo collecting is duplicates. Many negatives exist, so copies can be made. This is a big problem and because of it prices of photos are relatively low, $25 to $75.

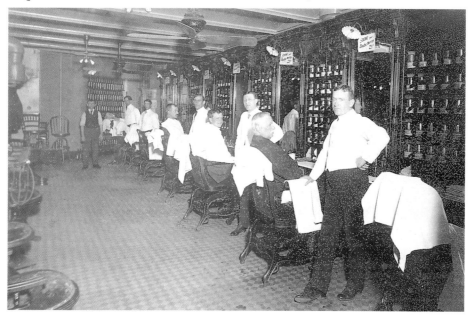

This photo shows several chairs and barbers. This is probably a large train station or hotel. There is a Central New York train sign in the rear. We see them advertising electric massage.

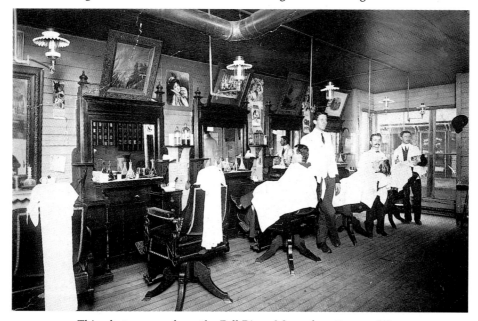

This photo comes from the Fall River, Massachusetts area. We can date this picture to 1903 because of the "Sarsaparilla" calendar. Also take note of the gas lighting and the mug rack reflection in back bar mirror.

Mug Racks

Authentic barber shop mug racks are difficult to find, especially the larger examples with over fifty holes. Racks that date from the 1890s usually have solid separators between mug compartments. Racks after this have a thin piece of wood as a separator. This would allow airflow throughout the rack shelf, keeping things dry and fungus free.

Racks found today are usually beat up and in need of repair. But there is a status in having an original rack. The mugs seem to show better when placed on the real thing. Prices for racks are determined by mug separator holes. Standard oak racks with little trim and around 30 holes sell for around $600, or about $20 per hole. Larger racks in walnut would be more, about $30 per hole. Shown here are examples from the catalog.

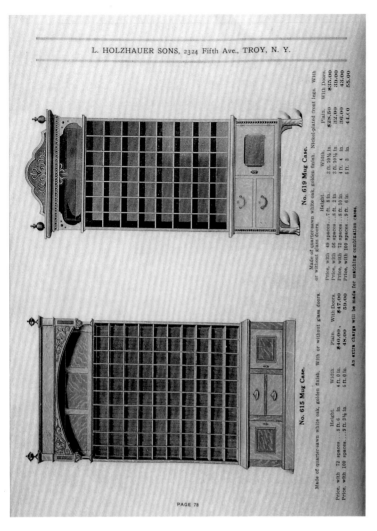

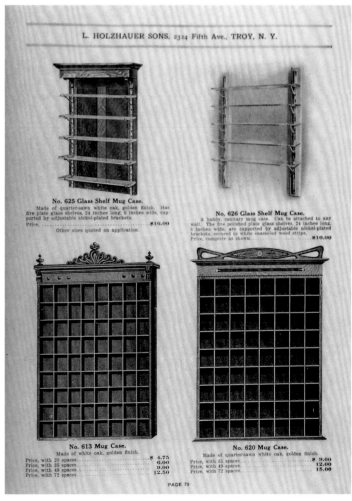

Barberiana

Bill and Phyllis Gilmore have created an 1900s barber shop in their home. Many items from several different shops have been brought together in one impressive collection. The red plush chair (1905) is from Koken Barber supply of St. Louis. The cash register is from a shop in Gahanna, Ohio, which was frequented by Bill when he was a youth. Other items such as hand painted barber poles and a sign from a Chillicothe, Ohio barber shop stating "If you leave the shop you lose your turn." Perhaps the most unique item is the Ever-Ready safety razor wooden pendulum clock. Mug racks from five different barber shops house Bill's collection.

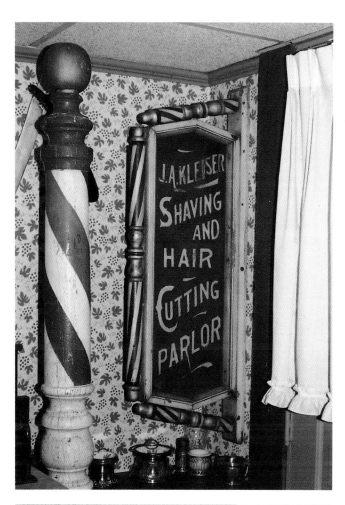

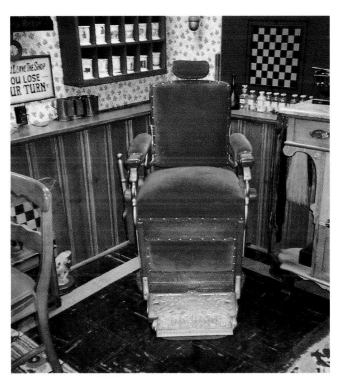

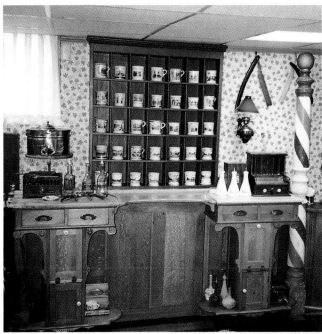

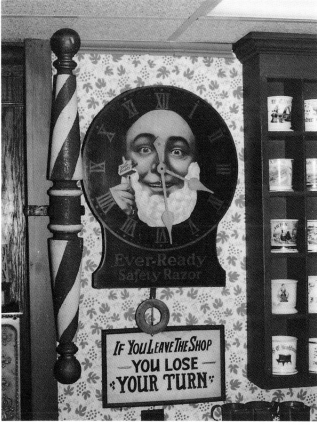

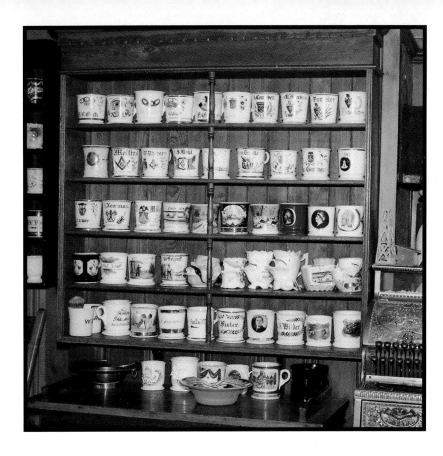

One of five mug racks used to house Bill's collection.

Clam Broth

Many mugs, bottles and other items were made obsolete in the 1920s with the popularity of American made Clam Broth glassware. These heavy bottles and items could take much more punishment than the art glass barber bottle. They're also a standard color, white, which became the new color for barber shop interiors. Many of these items are still in use today. The bottles are most numerous and worth $5-15. All other items, such as cream jars and sterilizer jars, are worth $25. Some mugs were still personalized and these are not easily found. I would price them $75 to $100. The most expensive item is the shaving paper vase worth $150 to $200. Some of these items can be fancy with silver overlays and are worth 50% more.

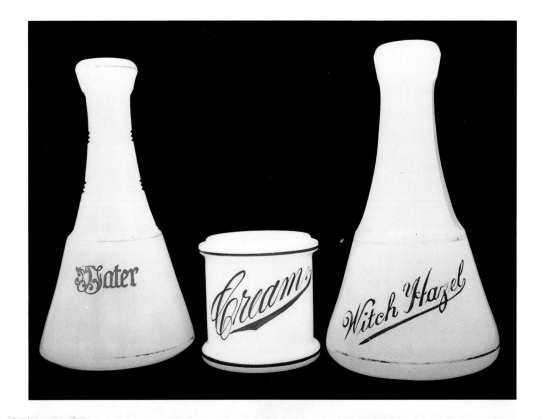

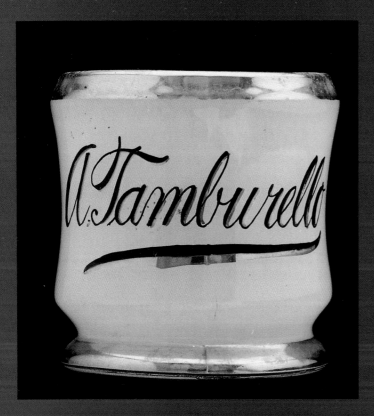

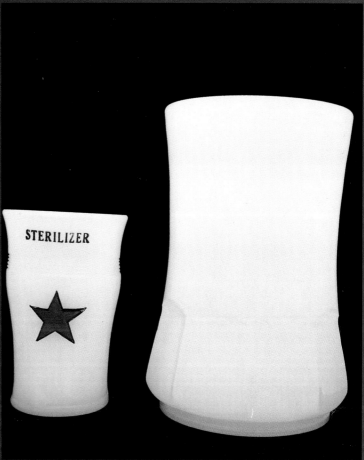

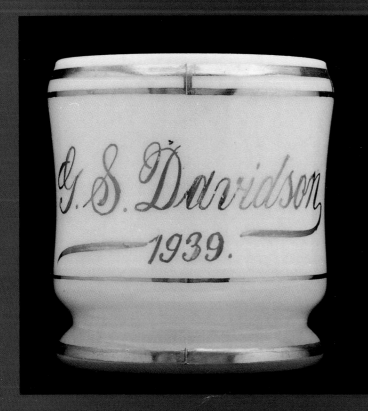

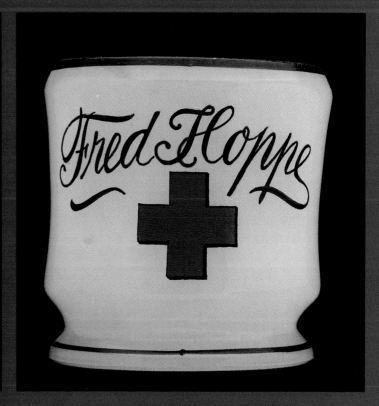

Chapter 7
Selling and Repairing Mugs

No one can tell you how to collect. As an individual you have your own ideas and goals. All mugs have value and there is no crystal ball which will allow you to see what mug prices will be in the future.

Here are a few tips, from my own experience. Florals and Decoratives will probably experience a sharp rise over the next five years- as more collectors come along. These are areas which are still relatively inexpensive.

Fraternals may provide the greatest gain. Fraternals with positive determining factors should double or triple in value over the next ten years. Why? Occupationals can cost $500 or $600 for a good collection grade example. Fraternals in good collection grade go for $125 to $200. When new collectors come along and find themselves priced out of the Occupational category, they will seek the next best alternative—quality Fraternals.

I have frequently been asked, "I can only spend $500 a year on my hobby. Should I buy several Florals and Decoratives or one Occupational?" The answer I give is that you should never fence yourself into a $500 limit. New collectors have beginner's luck, if you find a great Occupational for $400, but have already spent $400 on Decoratives, buy the Occupational anyway. The greatest mistake is passing on a mug that you should have bought. You are building wealth as well as a collection. New collectors seem to want to limit themselves, perhaps as justification to a spouse. If you have to, use next year's $500; you will come into low periods where you will not find mugs for months or even a year. Always take advantage of a good situation.

Selling Your Mugs

If you are selling your mugs you may be asking yourself a few questions. Should I get an appraisal? Are mugs with chips worth anything? Should I allow strangers into my house to see the mugs? My nephew's friend wants to buy two mugs, should I sell them?

The most important thing you can do is get an appraisal. It should be a written appraisal, not a ballpark figure. You should have it done by a professional antiques dealer who is familiar with barber shop items. If you have your collection appraised and the dealer offers to buy it for its appraised value, beware. Most appraisals are replacement values for insurance purposes. A dealer's mark up is usually 20% to 25%, a correct offer should be 75% to 80% of the appraised value.

Mugs with problems still have value. Sometimes it's about half the value of a perfect mug, providing that it is collection grade or better.

Allowing strangers into your house is a bad idea for anyone regardless of mug collecting. Someone may seem pleasant over the phone, but in your house he may become intimidating. You may become nervous and make a mistake by selling your mugs.

One of the worst mistakes you can make is allowing someone to "pick" your collection. In my experience as a dealer every collection has one or two mugs that are worth far more than any other in the collection. Sometimes two mugs can hold half the value of a twenty mug collection. By allowing someone to "pick," like your nephew's friend, you stand a chance of losing your best mugs, and your collection now has no interest to an advanced collector.

One more piece of important advice is never try to alter a mug. I would not even wash the mugs if they were dirty. A good one may slip from your hands and break.

If you are selling your mugs and bottles you should consider a private treaty sale. This is when your mug is appraised, and guaranteed to sell at a certain price. But the dealer will pursue a higher price on your behalf. The commission is usually lower than an auctioneer's. When you consign a mug for an auction it can take months for the auction date and sometimes it can take a while to be paid. A private treaty sale starts immediately and a successful sale could take place within a week.

Mug Damage and Repair

It amazes me that any hard-used piece of china could have survived intact over the last one hundred years.

First generation collectors could be selective, as the supply was plentiful in the 1950s and 60s. Even so, there were several who collected any mug they found, regardless of condition. In most cases, however, collectors would pass on mugs with excessive gold wear and damage.

With fierce competition among collectors today, damaged, repaired and regilded mugs are more commonly accepted. There is a set of determining factors for mugs with problems. Some damage is still considered unacceptable.

"Crack in the Making." This is a problem which doesn't detract any value from the mug. It's a common problem occurring where the top of the handle meets the main body of the mug.

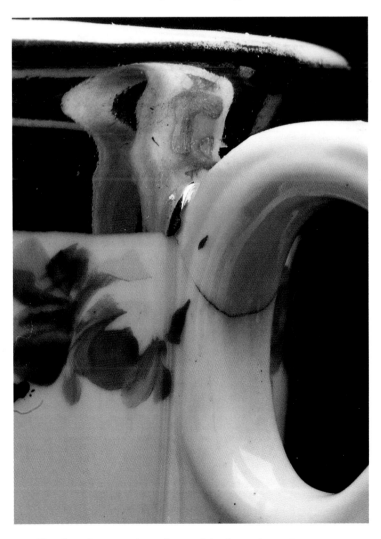

Here's a close-up view of a crack in the making. As you can see, this is a very minor flaw.

"Re-gilding." Gold loss is a very common problem and the repair is acceptable to the majority of collectors. There are two processes for re-gilding, "Cold Gold" and "Refired Gold."

The cold gold process is nothing more than a high quality gold paint which is applied to the mug. The problem with this method is that the gold has a mustard color and doesn't have a mirror finish.

Refired gold is basically doing what the original mug decorator did when applying somebody's name to a mug. A high quality gold is painted on the mug, then it is fired in the kiln. This process could have taken place a hundred years ago if the customer wanted his name reapplied to the mug. This particular process is not without problems. Sometimes an unseen fault may cause the mug to be damaged or break in the kiln. Another problem is that certain blanks will spot when they are reheated. Sometimes this spotting is very minor at other times it will ruin the appearance of the mug. Blanks of high quality, usually from France and Germany, refire with no problems. Semi-vitreous mugs can't be refired. The illustration shows what happens when this is attempted.

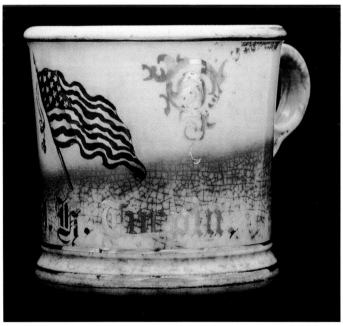

The effects of refiring a semi-vitreous mug.

Rim and Base Chips This is another common problem of the rim and base, which were the most exposed areas of the mug. If the barber's hands were wet and a mug slipped from them, the chances of a rim or base chip were great.

Except for gold refiring, all other repairs are done with a cold process. Base and rim chips are repaired with a cold filler and then painted to match the mug.

After fixing, any gold trim repair must use cold gold process, as a mug can't be refired with repaired chips. A chip repair to the rear of the mug is more desirable, as you will not see it when you're viewing the graphics.

Broken Handles. Broken handles are another common problem. Sometimes you will find a mug with a very crude, but solid repair. I believe these were damaged by the barber, and the original owner insisted that he have it repaired.

There are two ways to fix a broken handle. A small chip or break can be repaired in a way similar to a chip repair. A massive break, leaving only two stubs where the handle was, can be repaired by having the remainder ground or cut off. A good handle can be removed from a damaged or Gold Name mug and cut to fit the mug to be repaired.

Unacceptable Damage. Large, unsightly cracks are considered unacceptable, especially if they are in the graphics. It should be apparent by now that it is the folk art quality of the mug which makes it desirable. Any damage through the illustration affects the "art" of the mug. Only on extremely rare graphics would illustration damage be acceptable.

Perhaps the worst damage is the damage of "ignorance." When someone finds an old mug in an attic, they have an idea that it is of value and they intend to sell it. But before this person seeks the knowledge of an antiques dealer, they decide that nobody would want a mug with someone else's name. So they proceed to take the name off with steel wool or a Brillo pad. Along with the owner's name the top layer of glaze comes off and scratches are caused. A mug in this condition can't be refired. The new gold will run into the scratches when the mug is heated, and come out smudged. Only a cold repair can be done. The mug will never be acceptable to an advanced collector.

Before and After

Would you collect a repaired mug? Can you tell if you own one now? Here is a mug with a broken handle and 90% natural gold loss. Many collectors would pass on this mug, but not me. Why? Because it is a telephone lineman, and represents my industry—telecommunications.

The mug is first regilded then the old handle is completely removed. Another handle, in excellent condition is cut to fit perfectly. And we see the mug after its repair.

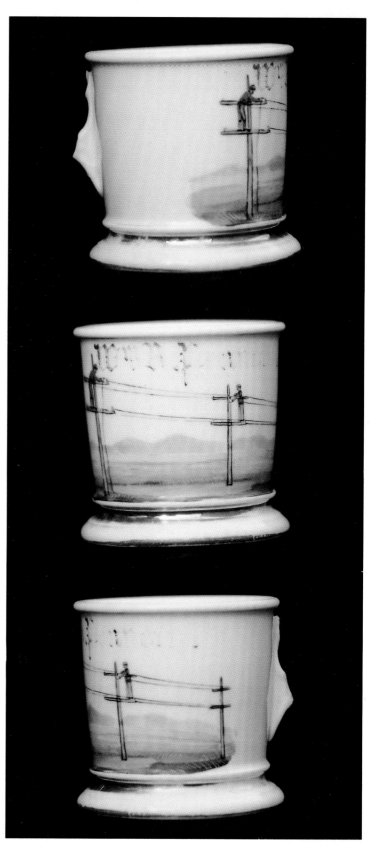

A mug in sorry shape, yet because the telephone lineman represents my industry, I want to add it to my collection.

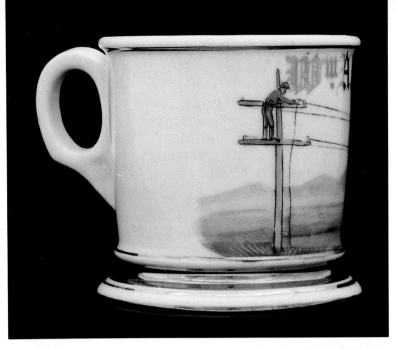

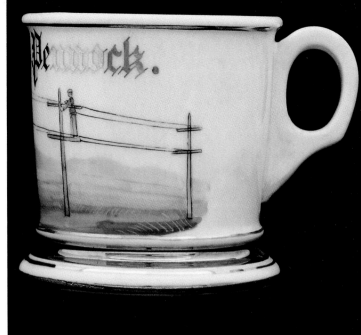

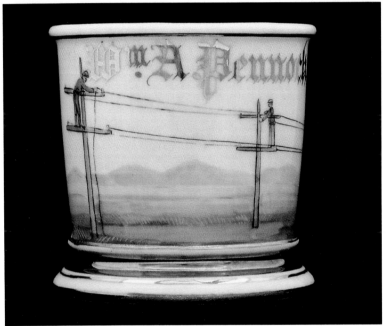

With high quality repairs it is a nice addition to my collection.

An Old Trick

Sometimes you will find a mug which has what you believe to be a repair. You may be hesitant to buy the mug, but the person selling it tells you that "it's nothing." To check it out, all you'll need is a small lamp, with the shade removed. Put the mug over the light bulb and turn it on. Fine old china will pass light and expose every fault the mug has.

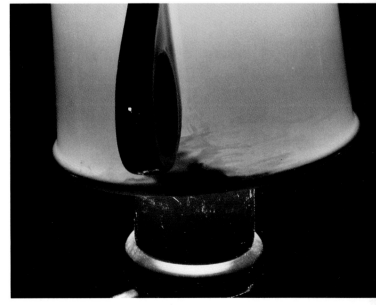

Here is an example of a mug put over a light bulb. Notice the area above the handle. This is what a cold chip repair looks like. No matter how good the repair may be, the light bulb will tell you the truth. This little trick doesn't work on semi-vitreous mugs because they are pottery and won't pass light.

Afterword

William R. Breit
1868-1924

Mr. Breit lived in Stratford and Sandy Hook, Connecticut. He owned the Connecticut Chain Company of Bridgeport. This company specialized in the manufacture of confectionery machines. The picture, mug and letterhead all date from around 1905.

The shaving mug is a common Floral design, which in no way represents the owner's occupation. In this case, the taffy cooling table or the buttercup cutter would have made a wonderful Occupational.

I only wish that my great grandfather had brought the letterhead to the barber shop and requested it as the design for his mug.

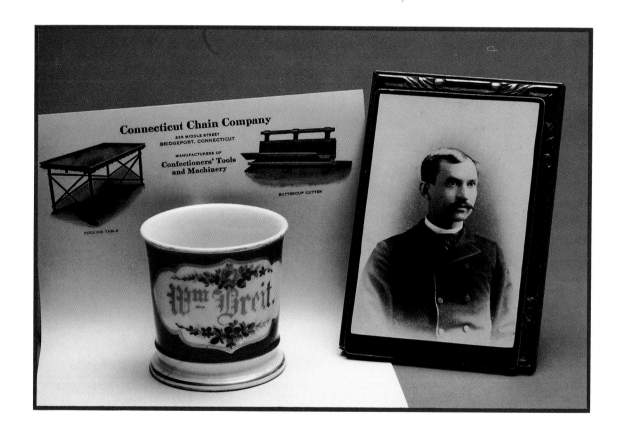

References

Barlow, Raymond E., and Joan E. Kaiser. *The Glass Industry in Sandwich, Volume 4.* Barlow-Kaiser Publishing, 1983.

Barlow, Ronald S. *The Vanishing American Barber Shop.* Windmill Publishing, 1993.

Griffin, Michael J., Editor. *Barber Shop Collecitbles News Letter.* A National Shaving Mug Collectors Association publication, 1986-Present.

Holiner, Richard. *Collecting Barber Bottles.* Collector Books, 1986.

Holtzhauer Barber Supplies Catalog, c. 1915.

Powell, Robert Blake. *Antique Shaving Mugs of the United States.* Self-published, 1972.

Powell, Robert Blake. *Occupational & Fraternal Shaving Mugs of the United States.* Self-published, 1978.

Ware, W. Porter. *Occupational Shaving Mugs.* Lightner Publishing Corporation, 1949.

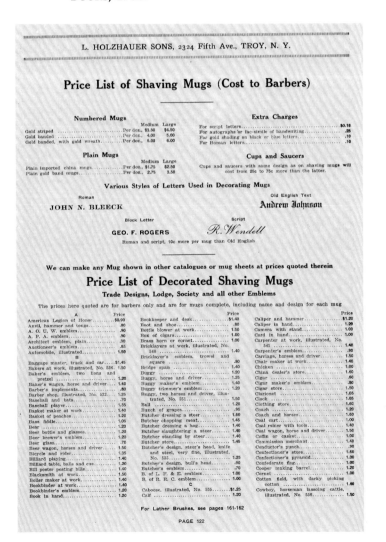

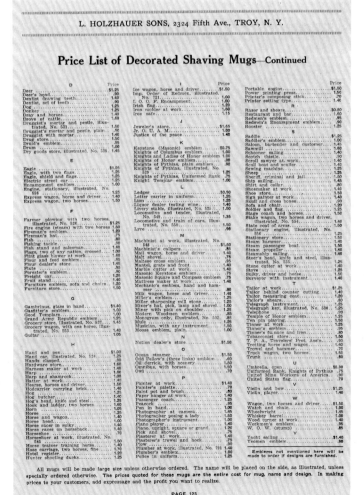

Price List of Decorated Shaving Mugs

Illustrated on pages 114 to 120 inclusive

The prices quoted below are for barbers only, and are for mugs complete, including name and design for each mug
A deposit is required with each order, if the full amount is not paid. See page 3 for terms.
The prices quoted are for designs as represented. If changes are ordered extra charge will have to be made

		Price
500	Autograph, or fac-simile of owner's handwriting	$0.75
501	Script letters	.50
502	Monogram	.85
513	Heavy gold band top and bottom	.60
520	Blacksmith with anvil and hammer	1.00
524	Railway hand-car, very natural	1.25
525	Livery stable, building, buggies, horses, etc.	1.50
526	Farmer plowing in field, houses, barns and scenery in distance	1.25
529	Knights of Pythias	1.25
530	Telegraph key	1.25
531	Druggist's mortar	1.50
532	Barber shop	1.25
535	Steer's head, knife and steel	1.25
536	Bakers at work	1.50
537	Grocery store	1.45
538	Dry goods store	1.45
540	Bricklayer at work	1.40
541	Carpenter at work	1.40
545	Horseshoer at work	1.50
548	Machinist at work	1.50
549	Locomotive and tender	1.25
550	Locomotive and train of cars	1.50
551	Man in buggy, with spanking double team	1.50
553	Grocery wagon, with one horse	1.40
554	Two-horse stake wagon	1.50
555	R. R. caboose	1.25
556	Stationary engine, very exact and complete	1.25
558	Cowboy, horseman lassoing cattle	1.50
568	Bluebird, ribbon and flowers, very attractive	1.00
625	Black ground, banded by ice fields top and bottom, gold base and handle	1.50

		Price
634	A. O. U. W. anchor and shield on an artistic fan with forget-me-not, white ribbon for name	$1.50
644	Brotherhood of R. R. Trainmen, showing lantern, red and green flags	1.25
658	Artistic winter landscape, showing bird sitting on branches in the foreground	.80
664	Ornamented gold band and sprays, with roses	1.00
667	New saloon design	1.45
701	Spray of roses	.50
704	American flag	1.00
708	Dog and snipe	1.15
710	Two horse heads	1.25
718	Knights of Pythias	.90
720	Woodmen of America	.85
721	Redmen's emblem	.90
723	Masonic square and compass emblem	.70
740	Two horses frightened by flash of lightning	1.50
748	Black background, white letters	1.00
754	Birds sitting on limb of a tree	.65
766	Elk's emblem; handsomely executed	.90
769	Woodmen of the World emblem, plain design	.85
771	F. O. E. emblem, eagle and cross flags, filigree	1.00
773	A neat bunch of violets and leaves under a well executed gold filigree	.60
783	Sweet peas, variously colored	.75
784	Hunter shooting birds, a pleasing design for a sportsman	1.25
785	Knights of Columbus emblem	1.00
786	Odd Fellow's 3-link emblem	.60
791	Plumber at work	1.40

		Price
796	A magnificent Elk emblem against the official Elk colors of purple and white, surrounded with heavy raised gold and forget-me-nots	$2.00
799	Two horses' heads in raised gold frame, surrounded by maroon background and flowers	2.00
800	Bird dogs, a work of art, in frame of embossed gold against blended background	2.00
802	White and pink tea roses, with richly blended background	1.00
803	Cowboy on galloping horse, a striking design in true western coloring	1.50
808	Carefully drawn dynamo, design of especial merit	1.50
809	Automobile	1.50
	Design of any special make can be furnished if supplied with a cut, also if furnished with a photo. We will transfer automobile with occupants to mug in an artistic manner	2.50
810	Elk's emblem; latest design	1.00
811	Masonic emblem, with blended blue background and gold filigree	1.20
812	A neat cluster of cherries	.70
813	Moose emblem, in blended maroon background	1.30
814	Spray of roses with green background	1.35
815	Scalloped forget-me-not design	1.25
816	Conventional violet design	1.25
817	Duck and drake design surrounded by a lake background	1.50
818	An attractive currant design with blended background	1.00
819	Groups of yellow roses with green shading	.90

238

VALUE GUIDE

Using This Guide

The values listed represent, in the opinion of the author, what an item *which is in excellent condition* might be valued at by the knowledgeable collector. Pieces illustrated may vary in condition, but are priced as Excellent. The price paid for any particular item will vary by geographical location, and will also be affected by the eagerness of the buyer, willingness of the seller, whether purchased at a retail shop, antique show, or flea market.

Items with excessive wear, chipping or breakage are worth less than the values listed.

Ultimately the price paid for any particular item depends on the buyer and seller. The author does not claim to be the final authority on prices and assumes no responsibility for financial loss or gain based on the use of this guide.

Position Codes

T = Top	TL = Top Left	BR = Bottom Right
C = Center	TC = Top Center	CL = Center left
B = Bottom	TR = Top Right	CR = Center right
R = Right	BL = Bottom Left	L = Left
	BC = Bottom Center	

Pg.	Pos.	Value
1	C	$150-200
2	TL	$300-350
2	TR	$100-175
3	B	$200-225
4	B	$250
6	B	$150
8	T	$20 ea.
12	TR	$225
14	BL	$100
17	TR	$100
17	CL	$25-50
17	CR	$15-35
18	TL	$25-35
18	TR	$25-35
18	BL	$200-250
18	BR	$200-250
19	TL	$150-200
19	TR	$75-125
19	BL	$75-150
19	BR	$60
20	TL	$75-125
20	TR	$150-175
20	BL	$150-175
20	BR	$25-35
21	CL	$75-125
21	CR	$100-200
21	BL	$200-400
21	BR	$150-300
22	TR	$200-300
22	B	$300-400
23	TR	$200-300
23	BL	$300-400
23	BR	$250-350
24	TR	$250-400
24	CL	$250-400
24	B	$150-200 set
25	TR	$1,000
25	CL	$75-150
25	CR	$300-400
25	BR	$150-200
26	TL	$150
26	CR	$50
26	BR	$100-200
27	TL	$500-700
27	TR	$450-550
27	BR	$1,000

Pg.	Pos.	Value
28	TL	$450-650
28	BL	$300-400
28	BR	$300-400
29	TR	$350-450
29	CL	$200-300
29	BR	$300-400
30	TL	$300-400
30	CL	$75-100
30	BR	$250-350
31	TR	$500-600
31	B	$400-600
32	BL	$75-125
33	TR	$125-175
33	CL	$175-250
33	BL	$300-400
33	BR	$250-350
34	CL top	$200-300
34	CL left	$75-150
34	CL right	$175-250
34	BR	$700-800
35	TR	$1,000+
35	CR	$800-1,000
35	BL	$700-800
36	TR	$500-700
36	CL	$450-650
36	BR	$1,000+
37	TR	$400-600
37	B	$800-$1,000
38	TR	$600-800
38	BR	$1,000+
39	CR	$125-175
42	CR	$20-25
42	BR	$20-30
43	TL	$25-35
43	TR	$25-35
43	BL	$25-35
43	BR	$25-50
44	TL	$35-60
44	CL	$25-35
44	CR	$30-50
44	BR	$25-40
45	TL	$35-65
45	CR	$35-65
45	BL	$40-70
46	TL	$35-50
46	CL	$35-50

Pg.	Pos.	Value
46	CR	$35-50
46	BR	$35-50
47	TL	$50-75
47	CL	$50-100
47	CR	$50-100
47	BR	$50-100
48	TL	$100-150
48	CL	$175-300
48	CR	$100-200
48	BL	$150-250
48	BR	$100-175
49	TL	$100-200
49	TR	$100-200
49	CL	$100-200
49	CR	$100-200
49	BL	$150-250
49	BR	$150-250
50	TL	$150-250
50	CR	$100-150
50	B	$125-175
51	TL	$100-150
51	TR	$125-150
51	CL	$100-150
51	CR	$200-250
51	BL	$150-175
51	BR	$100-150
52	TL	$150-175
52	TR	$200-300
52	CL	$150-200
52	CR	$200-300
52	BL	$175-275
52	BR	$200-300
53	T	$250-350
53	BL	$200-300
53	BR	$200-300
54	TL	$150-200
54	CL	$150-200
54	BR	$150-250
55	TL	$100-200
55	CR	$100-200
55	B	$100-200
56	TL	$100-200
56	TR	$150-200
56	CL	$175-250
56	CR	$175-250
56	BR	$150-250
57	TL	$150-250
57	TR	$200-400
57	CL	$250-300
57	CR	$200-400
57	BL	$100-200
57	BR	$150-300
58	TL	$250-300
58	TR	$250-300
58	CL	$250-300
58	CR	$300-350
58	BR	$150-250
59	TL	$100-200
59	TR	$150-250
59	CL	$100-200
59	CR	$100-200
59	BL	$100-200
60	TL	$125-225
60	TR	$250-300
60	CL	$250-300
60	CR	$250-400
60	BR	$125-225
61	TL	$150-200
61	TR	$75-125
61	CL	$150-200
61	BL	$150-250
61	BR	$75-125
62	TL	$150-200
62	TR	$100-125
62	CL	$100-200
62	CR	$150-200
62	BR	$175-250
63	TL	$75-100
63	TR	$150-200
63	CL	$75-100
63	CR	$150-200
63	BR	$400+
64	TL	$150-250

Pg.	Pos.	Value
64	TR	$175-250
64	CL	$100-125
64	CR	$100-125
64	BR	$150-200
65	TL	$100-125
65	CL	$150-175
65	CR	$125-150
65	BR	$200-350
66	TL	$125-175
66	TR	$175-200
66	CL	$125-175
66	CR	$200-250
66	BL	$125-175
66	BR	$150-175
67	TL	$175-250
67	TR	$350+
67	CL	$150-200
67	CR	$250-350
67	BL	$150-200
68	TL	$200-400
68	TR	$150-200
68	CL	$150-200
68	CR	$150-200
68	BL	$250-300
68	BR	$250-300
69	TL	$300-400
69	TR	$300-400
69	CL	$300-400
69	CR	$300-500
69	BL	$250-350
69	BR	$300-500
70	TL	$75-150
70	TR	$75-150
70	BL	$75-150
70	BR	$75-150
71	TL	$75-150
71	CL	$300-450
71	CR	$350-500
71	BL	$300-450
71	BR	$350-500
72	TL	$250-325
72	TR	$1,000+
72	BL	$300-400
72	BR	$300-400
73	T	$300-400
73	B	$175-300
74	TL	$175-300
74	TR	$175-300
74	BL	$175-300
74	BR	$200-400
75	TL	$200-400
75	TR	$300-500
75	B	$250-350
76	TL	$250-350
76	TR	$350-600
76	CL	$400-600
76	CR	$350-600
76	BL	$250-400
76	BR	$1,000+
77	TL	$450-700
77	CL	$400-600
77	CR	$400-600
77	BL	$450-650
77	BR	$600-700
78	TL	$500-700
78	TR	$500-700
78	CL	$500-700
78	CR	$200-400
78	BL	$1,000+
78	BR	$200-400
79	TR	$250-450
79	CL	$250-450
79	CR	$600-800
79	BL	$350-500
79	BR	$600-800
80	TL	$350-550
80	TR	$400-600
80	B	$400-600
81	TL	$400-600
81	TR	$400-600
81	CL	$400-600
81	CR	$300-500
81	BL	$100-175
81	BR	$300-500

Pg.	Pos.	Value
82	TL	$600-800
82	TR	$600-800
82	CL	$350-650
82	CR	$600-800
82	BR	$800-1,000
83	TL	$1,000+
83	TR	$250-400
83	CR	$500-750
83	BL	$250-400
83	BR	$500-750
84	TL	$500-750
84	TR	$1,000+
84	CL	$1,000+
84	CR	$500-800
84	BL	$250-400
85	TL	$350-650
85	TR	$350-650
85	BR	$350-650
86	TL	$350-650
86	CL	$400-600
86	CR	$250-400
86	BR	$250-400
87	T	$350-500
87	BL	$600-800
87	BR	$500-700
88	TL	$500-700
88	TR	$600-800
88	CL	$450-650
88	CR	$600-800
88	BL	$500-700
88	BR	$600-800
89	TL	$800-1,000
89	TR	$1,000+
89	CL	$400-650
89	CR	$800-1,000
89	BL	$500-700
89	BR	$650-850
90	T	$600-800
90	B	$200-300
91	TL	$400-500
91	TR	$400-500
91	CL	$600-750
91	CR	$250-400
91	BL	$600-75
91	BR	$1,000+
92	TL	$800-1,000
92	TR	$250-300
92	B	$400-500
93	T	$250-350
93	BL	$400-600
93	BR	$400-600
94	TL	$400-600
94	TR	$850-1,000
94	CL	$500-700
94	BL	$850-1,000
94	BR	$300-400
95	TL	$300-400
95	TR	$700-900
95	CL	$400-550
95	BL	$600-700
95	BR	$250-400
96	TL	$350-600
96	TR	$400-600
96	CL	$800-1,000
96	CR	$350-650
96	BR	$1,000+
97	TL	$600-800
97	TR	$350-550
97	CL	$800-1,000
97	CR	$400-600
97	BL	$600-800
97	BR	$700-1,000
98	TL	$800-1,000
98	TR	$500-700
98	CL	$750-1,000
98	CR	$500-800
98	BL	$600-800
98	BR	$600-800
99	TL	$1,000
99	TR	$600-800
99	CL	$700-800
99	CR	$800-1,000
99	BL	$600-750

Pg.	Pos.	Value
99	BR	$1,000+
100	TL	$1,000+
100	TR	$250-400
100	CL	$1,000+
100	CR	$300-400
100	BL	$750-850
100	BR	$500-700
101	TL	$200-300
101	TR	$250-350
101	BL	$300-400
101	BR	$200-300
102	TL	$200-300
102	TR	$600-800
102	CR	$600-800
102	BL	$600-800
102	BR	$800-1,000
103	TL	$1,000+
103	TR	$750-1,000
103	CL	$1,000+
103	BL	$750-1,000
103	BR	$750-1,000
104	TL	$750-1,000
104	TR	$750-1,000
104	CL	$750-1,000
104	BL	$750-1,000
104	BR	$1,000+
105	TR	$750-1,000
105	CL	$1,000+
105	CR	$750-1,000
105	BL	$750-1,000
105	BR	$500-700
106	TR	$600-800
106	CL	$600-800
106	CR	$800-1,000
106	BL	$550-750
106	BR	$400-600
107	TL	$400-600
107	TR	$300-400
107	BL	$350-450
107	BR	$1,000+
108	T	$200-350
108	BL	$200-350
108	BR	$400-600
109	T	$400-600
109	BL	$400-600
109	BR	$400-600
110	TL	$400-600
110	TR	$250-350
110	CR	$600-800
110	BL	$400-600
110	BR	$650-850
111	TL	$800-1,000
111	TR	$1,000+
111	CL	$500-750
111	CR	$1,000+
111	BL	$650-800
111	BR	$1,000+
112	TL	$1,000+
112	TR	$600-800
112	CR	$600-800
112	BL	$600-800
112	BR	$600-800
113	TL	$600-800
113	TR	$800-1,000
113	CL	$1,000+
113	CR	$800-1,000
113	BR	$1,000+
114	TL	$250-300
114	TR	$250-300
114	B	$250-350
115	T	$250-350
115	BL	$300-400
115	BR	$300-400
116	TL	$350-550
116	TR	$350-450
116	CL	$300-500
116	CR	$350-550
116	BL	$1,000+
116	BR	$400-600
117	TL	$400-600
117	CR	$400-600
117	BL	$350-450
118	T	$300-500
118	CL	$300-500

Pg.	Pos.	Value	Pg.	Pos.	Value	Pg.	Pos.	Value	Pg.	Pos.	Value	Pg.	Pos.	Value	Pg.	Pos.	Value
118	CR	$400-700	136	TR	$300-500	155	TR	$500-700	178	BR	$20	204	BR right	$175	231	TR left	$25
118	B	$400-700	136	CL	$250-350	155	CL	$600-800	179	T	$10-20 ea.	205	TR	$150 ea.	231	TR right	$150
119	TL	$1,000+	136	CR	$400-600	155	BL	$500-700	179	BL	$25-50	205	BL left	$300	231	BL	$75
119	TR	$450-750	136	BR	$500-700	155	BR	$800-1,000	179	BR	$25-50	205	BL right	$150	231	BR	$75
119	CL	$600-800	137	TL	$600-700	156	TL	$800-1,000	180	T	$100-200	206	TR	$175 ea.	235		$250
119	BL	$600-800	137	TR	$1,000+	156	TR	$2,000	180	B	$25-50	206	CL	$125 ea.			
119	BR	$800-1,000	137	CL	$600-700	156	CL	$800-1,000	181	T	$25-50	206	BR left	$100			
120	TL	$300-500	137	CR	$800-1,000	156	CR	$1,000+	181	C	$35-65	206	BR right	$125			
120	CL	$350-500	137	BL	$800-1,000	156	BR	$2,000+	181	B	$20 ea.	207	TL left	$400			
120	CR	$300-500	137	BR	$500-700	157	TL	$2,000+	182	T	$20-30 ea.	207	TL right	$200			
120	BR	$500-750	138	TL	$1,000+	157	TR	$1,500+	182	B	$20 ea.	207	CR left	$250			
121	TL	$800-1,000	138	TR	$800-1,000	157	CR	$1,000+	183	CL	$35-50	207	CR right	$500			
121	TR	$800-1,000	138	CL	$300-500	157	BL	$750-1,000	183	BR	$75-100	207	BL left	$450			
121	CL	$800-1,000	138	CR	$800-1,000	157	BR	$1,500+	184	B	$50 ea.	207	BL right	$350			
121	CR	$800-1,000	138	BL	$350-550	158	TL	$1,000+	185	TL	$100	208	TL left	$500			
121	BL	$400-600	138	BR	$1,000	158	CL	$1,000+	185	TR	$100+	208	TL right	$400			
121	BR	$1,000+	139	TL	$400-600	158	CR	$1,500+	185	BR	$100-150	208	BR	$550 ea.			
122	TL	$800-1,000	139	TR	$1,000+	158	BR	$1,500+	186	C	$10 ea.	209	TL left	$500			
122	TR	$600-750	139	CL	$600-800	159	TL	$1,000+	186	B	$25 ea.	209	TL right	$350			
122	CL	$800-1,000	139	CR	$750-1,000	159	CL	$500-700	187	T	$25 ea.	209	BR	$700 set			
122	CR	$800-1,000	139	BL	$300-400	159	BL	$2,000+	189	BL	$100	210	TL left	$175			
122	BL	$1,000+	139	BR	$750-1,000	159	BR	$2,000+	189	BR	$100	210	TL right	$125			
122	BR	$750-900	140	TL	$600-700	160	TR	$400-600	190	T	$600-800	210	BR	$300 set			
123	TL	$1,000	140	TR	$500-700	160	CL	$400-500	190	B	$250-500	211	L	$150			
123	TR	$500-750	140	B	$250-300	160	BR	$400-600	191	CR	$1,500+	211	R	$125			
123	B	$650-850	141	TL	$500-700	161	CL	$400-600	191	BL	$1,000+	212	TR	$150 ea.			
124	TL	$200-350	141	TR	$600-800	161	TR	$500-700	192	TL	$100-200 ea.	212	BL	$150 ea.			
124	TR	$400-600	141	CR	$1,000+	161	CR	$500-700	192	BL	$250-300 ea.	213	TL	$275 set			
124	CL	$200-350	141	BL	$600-800	161	BL	$500-700	194	TL	$175 ea.	213	CR	$250 ea.			
124	CR	$250-300	141	BR	$200-350	162	TL	$600-800	194	TR	$225 ea.	213	BL	$200 ea.			
124	BL	$350-550	142	TL	$400-600	162	TR	$600-800	194	BL left	$175	214	TL	$350 set			
125	TL	$300-400	142	TR	$400-600	162	BL	$600-800	194	BL right	$150	214	BR	$800-1,000 set			
125	TR	$600-800	142	CR	$400-600	162	BR	$500-700	194	BR	$150 ea.	215	TL	$750 ea.			
125	CL	$400-600	142	BL	$600-800	163	TL	$600-800	195	L	$225	215	BR	$750 ea.			
125	CR	$700-800	142	BR	$400-600	163	TR	$650-850	195	R	$150	216	L	$450			
125	BL	$500-750	143	TR	$350-500	163	BL	$500-700	196	TL left	$150	216	R	$250			
125	BR	$1,000+	143	CL	$350-500	163	BR	$700-900	196	TL right	$175	217	TL	$500 set			
126	TL	$600-800	143	BR	$600-700	164	TL	$800-1,000	196	TR left	$175	217	TR	$500 set			
126	TR	$500-700	144	T	$250-350	164	TR	$600-800	196	TR right	$150	217	BL	$200 ea.			
126	CL	$500-700	144	BL	$400-600	164	BL	$600-800	196	BL left	$100	217	BR	$500 set			
126	BR	$800-1,000	144	BR	$500-750	164	BR	$700-800	196	BL right	$150	218	TR	$525 set			
127	TR	$800-1,000	145	TL	$500-750	165	TL	$1,000+	196	BR left	$90	218	CL	$200 ea.			
127	CL	$1,000+	145	TR	$700-1,000	165	TR	$1,000+	196	BR right	$150	218	BR	$200 ea.			
127	CR	$400-600	145	CL	$500-750	165	BL	$800-1,000	197	TL left	$400	219	TL left	$200			
127	BL	$300-400	145	CR	$700-1,000	165	BR	$500-700	197	TL right	$150	219	TL right	$225			
128	TL	$400-600	145	BL	$500-750	166	TL	$650-850	197	CR left	$200	219	TR left	$300			
128	TR	$800-1,000	146	T	$1,000+	166	TR	$1,000+	197	CR right	$150	219	TR right	$275			
128	CL	$500-700	146	B	$1,000+	166	CL	$650-850	197	BL	$250 set	219	BL	$300 ea.			
128	BR	$300-400	147	T	$300-500	166	BR	$650-850	198	TR left	$125	219	BR left	$300			
129	TL	$750-900	147	BL	$500-700	167	TL	$650-850	198	TR right	$150	219	BR right	$275			
129	TR	$400-600	147	BR	$500-700	167	TR	$1,000+	198	CL left	$100	220	TR	$1,000+			
129	CL	$400-600	148	TL	$1,000+	167	BL	$700-900	198	CL right	$175	220	CL	$800+			
129	CR	$500-700	148	TR	$1,000+	167	BR	$700-900	198	BR left	$175	220	BR	$800+			
129	BL	$250-350	148	CL	$600-800	168	T	$150-175	198	BR right	$150	221	TL	$800+			
129	BR	$350-450	148	CR	$600-800	168	B	$200-225	199	TL left	$150	221	CR	$800+			
130	TL	$400-700	148	BL	$500-700	169	TL	$200-225	199	TL right	$175	221	BL	$800+			
130	TR	$250-350	148	BR	$1,000+	169	TR	$150-200	199	CR leftft	$100	222	TL	$600+			
130	CL	$350-450	149	TL	$1,000+	169	CL	$275-300	199	CR right	$75	222	BR	$800+			
130	CR	$400-600	149	CR	$1,500+	169	CR	$175-200	199	BL left	$125	223		$400-600			
130	BL	$250-300	149	BL	$1,000+	169	BL	$175-225	199	BL right	$250	224	TL	$100-125			
130	BR	$400-600	149	BR	$250-500	170	TL	$200-225	200	TR left	$100	225	Labels	$10 ea.			
131	T	$400-600	150	T	$600-800	170	TR	$400-450	200	TR right	$125	225	BR	$100			
131	BL	$500-700	150	BL	$600-800	170	BL	$350-400	200	CL left	$150	226	TL left	$100			
131	BR	$400-600	150	BR	$250-300	170	BR	$425-450	200	CL right	$175	226	TL right	$75			
132	TL	$300-400	151	TL	$250-300	171	TL	$200-250	200	BR	$175 ea.	226	TR	$75			
132	TR	$1,000+	151	TR	$250-350	171	CR	$175-200	201	TL left	$100	226	BL	$100			
132	CL	$800-1,000	151	CL	$300-400	171	B	$500	201	TL right	$150	226	BR	$75			
132	CR	$1,000+	151	BL	$300-400	172	T	$250-300	201	CR	$100 ea.	227	C	$50			
132	BR	$400-600	151	BR	$250-350	172	B	$275-325	201	BL	$275 ea.	227	B	$50			
133	TL	$800-1,000	152	TL	$300-400	173	T	$175-200 ea.	202	TR left	$400	229	TR sign	$500			
133	TR	$400-600	152	TR	$250-350	173	BL	$150-200	202	TR right	$350	229	TR pole	$800			
133	CL	$400-600	152	CR	$250-350	173	BR	$200-250	202	CL left	$150	229	CL chair	$800-1,000			
133	CR	$500-700	152	BL	$250-350	174	TL	$175-200	202	CL right	$125	229	BL rack	$750			
133	BL	$750-1,000	152	BR	$250-350	174	CR	$300-350	202	BR left	$375	229	BR clock	$800-1,000			
133	BR	$500-700	153	TL	$600-800	174	BL	$600-800	202	BR right	$300	229	BR sign	$300-500			
134	TL	$1,000+	153	TR	$700-800	175	TL	$600-800	203	TL left	$100	229	BR pole	$250			
134	TR	$1,000+	153	CL	$700-800	175	TR	$600-800	203	TL right	$150	230	TL	$500			
134	CL	$1,000+	153	CR	$300-400	175	BL	$600-800	203	CR	$250 ea.	230	B left	$10			
134	CR	$1,000+	153	BL	$700-800	175	BR	$600-800	203	BL left	$150	230	B center	$25			
134	BR	$500-700	153	BR	$600-800	176	TL	$250-300	203	BL right	$125	230	B right	$10			
135	TL	$500-700	154	T	$350-650	176	CL	$500-700	204	TL	$300 ea.	231	TL	$75			
135	TR	$1,500+	154	BL	$350-500	176	BR	$500-700	204	TR	$150 ea.						
135	B	$500-700	154	BR	$500-700	177		$1,000+	204	BL	$300 ea.						
136	TL	$100-150	155	TL	$500-700	178	BL	$10	204	BR left	$300						

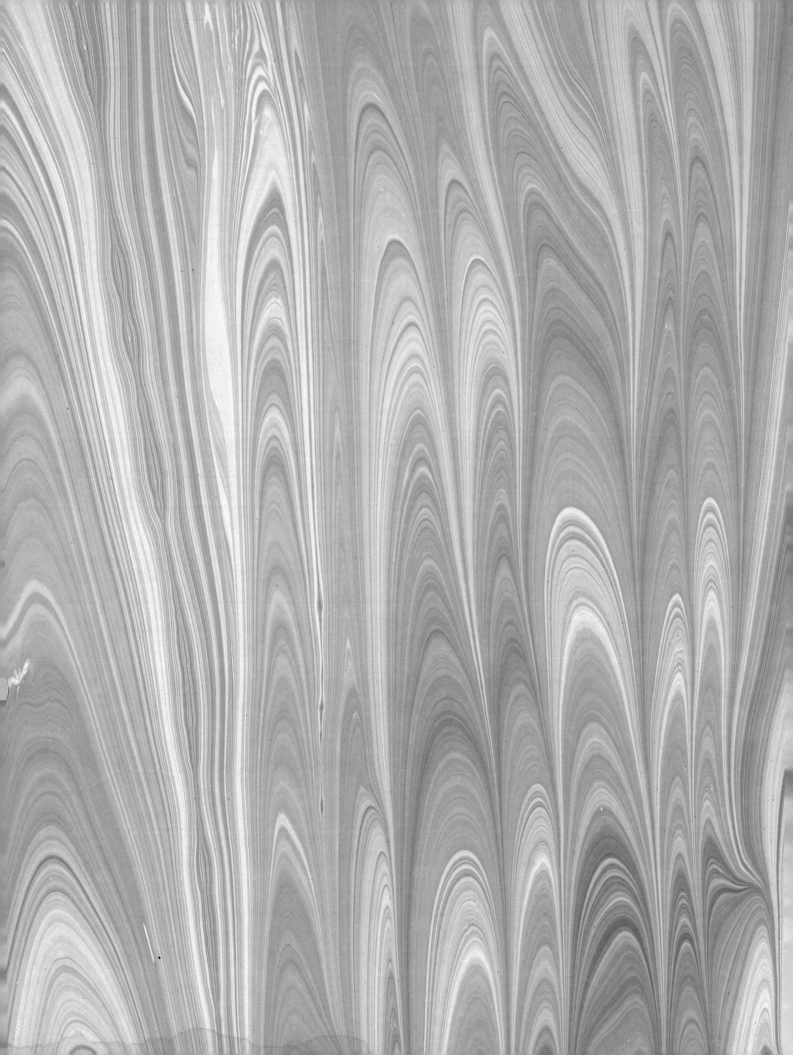